Risk and Crisis Communication During the COVID-19 Pandemic

This book examines the challenges of communicating messages during the COVID-19 pandemic and provides recommendations for managing future global health crises.

Given that outbreaks, epidemics, and pandemics are global crises that require global solutions, the book suggests that the world community needs to build resilient crisis management institutions and message management systems. Through international case studies, in-depth interviews, and textual, content, narrative, and document analysis, the book provides comprehensive accounts of how normative risk communication strategies were invoked, applied, disrupted, questioned, and changed during the COVID-19 pandemic. It explores themes including crisis preparedness, outbreak communication, lockdown messages, communication uncertainty, risk message strategies, and the challenges of information disorders. It argues that trust in supranational and national institutions is crucial for the effective management of future global public health crises.

A thorough assessment of the multiple challenges faced by public health authorities and audiences during the COVID-19 pandemic, this book will be of interest to researchers, practitioners, and students in the fields of Risk, Crisis, and Health Communication and Public Health and Disaster Management.

Martin N. Ndlela is a Professor of Crisis Communication at Inland Norway University of Applied Sciences, Norway, and Research Associate at the Department of Strategic Communication, University of Johannesburg.

Routledge Research in Communication Studies

Risk and Crisis Communication During the COVID-19 Pandemic

Muddled Messages

Martin N. Ndlela

Routledge
Taylor & Francis Group

NEW YORK AND LONDON

First published 2024
by Routledge
605 Third Avenue, New York, NY 10158

and by Routledge
4 Park Square, Milton Park, Abingdon, Oxon, OX14 4RN

Routledge is an imprint of the Taylor & Francis Group, an informa business

Library of Congress Cataloging-in-Publication Data
Names: Ndlela, Martin N., author.
Title: Risk and crisis communication during the COVID-19 pandemic : muddled messages / Martin N. Ndlela.
Other titles: Routledge research in communication studies.
Description: New York, NY : Routledge, 2024. | Series: Routledge research in communication studies | Includes bibliographical references and index.
Identifiers: LCCN 2023022656 (print) | LCCN 2023022657 (ebook) | ISBN 9781032513577 (paperback) | ISBN 9781032513560 (hardback) | ISBN 9781003401827 (ebook)
Subjects: MESH: Health Communication | COVID-19 | Emergencies | Health Information Management | Infodemic
Classification: LCC RA644.C67 (print) | LCC RA644.C67 (ebook) | NLM WA 590 | DDC 614.5/924144014—dc23/eng/20230607
LC record available at https://lccn.loc.gov/2023022656
LC ebook record available at https://lccn.loc.gov/2023022657

ISBN: 9781032513560 (hbk)
ISBN: 9781032513577 (pbk)
ISBN: 9781003401827 (ebk)

DOI: 10.4324/9781003401827

Typeset in Times New Roman
by codeMantra

Contents

1   The COVID-19 Pandemic

Introduction: "Communicate with Your People about the Risks"

The coronavirus disease 2019 (COVID-19), an infectious disease caused by the novel Severe Acute Respiratory Syndrome Coronavirus 2 (SARS CoV-2), appeared in China in late 2019, spread across the world like wildfire, and was later declared a pandemic by the World Health Organization (WHO). Since early 2020, public health authorities have battled to stop the scourge with mixed results. Some experts have even pondered over the possibility of COVID-19 becoming an endemic disease. The coronavirus pandemic has just shown how vulnerable humanity is to unexpected crises and how, in a connected world, what happens on some distant shores can produce local impacts, with far-reaching ramifications. To most countries in Africa, Europe, and South and North America, the outbreak of COVID-19 in China seemed remote, at least geographically. Given the history of coronavirus outbreaks, this was hardly an issue of major concern for most governments, oblivious to the fact that in an increasingly globalized world, there was a high risk of faster human-to-human transmission through air transport connections (Ndlela, 2021). The coronavirus pandemic appears to have arisen suddenly, even though antecedent signs were there for some months. As Lerbinger (1997) aptly describes this kind of crisis that builds up over time until a threshold is reached: "When this build-up is gradual and small, managers may be unaware of an approaching crisis, much as a frog placed in water that is very gradually heated, is unaware that it is about to be cooked to death". Health authorities around the world could not foresee that what was happening in China would soon engulf and affect everyone. Outbreaks occur often, but most of them retreat quickly without public notice. As the health crisis unfolded at the source of the outbreak, people across the world watched the drama live on media and social media. They watched in disbelief when on 22 January 2020, the central government in China imposed a complete lockdown on the epicentre, Wuhan, a city of 11 million people, and the other neighbouring cities in the populous Hubei province. It seemed baffling that a government would quarantine millions of people over an outbreak. The representative of the WHO

DOI: 10.4324/9781003401827-1

in China, Gauden Galea, described the move as unprecedented: "the lockdown of 11 million people is unprecedented in public health history, so it is certainly not a recommendation the WHO has made" (Reuters, 2020). In his comments, Galea also recognized the important decision taken by the Chinese authorities to contain the epidemic in the place where it was concentrated. Naturally, the happenings in China drew the attention of the media, which started to ponder on the gravity of the situation, the source and nature of the virus, mortality rates, and the practicalities of locking down a populous region. It wouldn't be long before the practice of lockdowns became a norm as authorities worldwide battled the coronavirus in their backyards for nearly two years.

On 11 March 2020, WHO declared COVID-19 a pandemic, based on the number of infections in more than 110 countries and territories around the world. In declaring the coronavirus a pandemic, WHO signalled a highest level of severity and threat posed by the virus to global public health. Declaring the COVID-19 outbreak a pandemic, WHO called for a "whole-of-government, whole-of-society approach" built around a comprehensive strategy to prevent infections, save lives, and minimize impact. This strategy entails extensive collaboration between public health authorities and private and humanitarian organizations. Above all, the global response calls for risk and crisis communication efforts to promote COVID-19 preventive behaviours and to mitigate the effects of the pandemic. WHO's clarion call was loud and clear:

Communicate with your people about the risks and how they can protect themselves.

This call forms the basis of this book, which seeks to explore the global challenges of risk and crisis communication messages during the COVID-19 pandemic. This book proceeds from a presumption that in a pandemic, public health information is a prerequisite tool for containing the spread of deadly diseases in the absence of any known medication. Providing public information messages timely and efficiently enables people at risk to make informed choices and actions to mitigate the effects of the crisis (Coombs, 2009; Sellnow, Lane, Sellnow, & Littlefield, 2017). Given the global nature of the pandemic risk and its implications, this book takes a global cross-cultural perspective on pandemic messages. Globalization, especially the increasing international movement of people, animals, and goods, is intricately linked with the increasing vulnerabilities of pandemic risks. As Carroll aptly puts it, "a threat anywhere is a threat everywhere" (quoted in French, 2022). "A pathogen originating in a poultry flock or a goat herd in a remote village in Africa or Asia can reach major cities on all continents within 36 hours" (Jonas, 2013, p. 12). In a globalized world, no country is an island, and capacities of public health systems and their communication capabilities have ramifications beyond national boundaries. Given that the pandemic risk is shared globally, local and national public health authorities are expected to co-ordinate their tasks and communicate messages with international stakeholders.

This book locates the challenges within two major developments in public health communications that have impacted heavily on the pandemic communications and shaped the reception and acceptance of risk and crisis communication messages during the pandemic.

First, the pandemic is unique, in that it is the first pandemic to occur in an era of widespread artificial intelligence (AI) and algorithm-driven digital communications. These technological developments have had a profound influence on communication, impacting the production, dissemination, and consumption of pandemic messages. The technologies enabled an unprecedented massive production and consumption of both filtered and unfiltered information about the pandemic. The declining role of the mass media as information gatekeepers and the increase in user-generated content saw a preponderance of false information, disinformation, and rumours during the pandemic period. Users taking advantage of AI combined with social media vulnerability contributed to the falsification of the public sphere (Santini, Salles, Tucci, Ferreira, & Grael, 2020). Given the pervasiveness of social media manipulation and computational propaganda (Santini et al., 2020), WHO bemoaned the negative impact of the infodemic, that is, too much false or misleading information in the digital and physical environment during a disease outbreak, on pandemic information messages. Infodemics undoubtedly have implications on the reception and understanding of pandemic information messages and consequently on the citizens' knowledge of the risks and their ability to protect themselves.

Second, the pandemic took place in a period where "trust appeared to be under threat everywhere" (Pond, 2020) and in an era characterized by the rise of a post-truth culture where objective facts are less influential in shaping public opinion. In this era, as Pond (2020) posits, "nobody knows anything anymore" and "truth is irrelevant". Within this context characterized by the crisis of trust and the rise of post-truth politics, public health authorities had to grapple with sceptical audiences, the phenomena of science denialism and its harm to pandemic messages. Public understanding of science is crucial for the reception of messages and adhering to science-based recommendations. The infodemic compounded the crisis of trust and arguably undermined the communication of risks to the public. It undermined trust in the messages and in the messengers. Sinatra and Hofer (2021) note how:

> pronouncing the novel coronavirus pandemic a hoax or dismissing the effects of COVID-19 as no more problematic than the flu has led to the loss of many lives, especially when those erroneous beliefs led to policies that failed to protect citizens.

(p. 9)

During the pandemic, people, including prominent public figures, died from COVID-19 still questioning science, in denial and in doubt about the risk it posed to their lives. The unwillingness to change one's mind considering the evidence about the risk posed by the coronavirus hinges on the prevailing attitude towards science and trust in public health institutions. Taken together with the availability of an enormous amount of information on digital platforms and the easiness to falsify evidence compounded the situation leading vulnerable citizens to disregard otherwise useful messages.

Trust is fundamental in message reception, yet we have seen some countries struggling to communicate with their citizens due to diminishing levels of trust in the mass media and public institutions. Trust is very vital in situations that are difficult to understand (Boin, 't Hart, Stern, & Sundelius, 2016; Sellnow & Seeger, 2021), and the COVID-19 pandemic created a need for trust in science, government, and state agencies. Multiple studies show that people who trust in science are more likely to comply with official guidelines (Bicchieri et al., 2021; Sulik et al., 2021). Research in the Nordic countries has highlighted how the higher levels of institutional trust positively impacted pandemic communications, increasing levels of citizens' compliance with protective measures (Johansson, Ihlen, Lindholm, & Blach-Ørsten, 2023). Conversely, lack of trust negatively affects risk perception, thereby obstructing citizens' willingness to comply with risk mitigation measures (Johnsson, Solhberg, & Esaiasson, 2023).

Public Health Risk

Risk is a diffuse concept that can mean different things to different people. Risk is defined as "future events that may occur, that threaten us" (Beck, 2009, p. 9). A public health risk is defined as something likely to be harmful to human health. When a public health risk becomes manifest, a crisis can occur (Coombs, 2023). The probability that an undesirable disease outbreak, situation, or condition will occur was anything but evident. Global concern about the pandemic threat has always been there. The salient characteristic of the pandemic is that it combines a low probability of occurring with a high, potentially catastrophic, global impact (Jonas, 2013). The outbreak of a highly infectious coronavirus posed a threat to human health, economies, and communities. Respiratory infections are often highly transmissible, and they are easy to transmit from an infected person to several other people within a short period. The WHO expressed deep concern about the "alarming levels of spread and severity" of the coronavirus (WHO, 2020: n.pag.). It was spreading fast and posed a formidable threat to global society as a whole.

When a public health risk is identified and assessed, actions are taken to either eliminate or reduce it to a reasonable level (Coombs, 2023; Levitt, 1997). Once a pandemic is underway, its impact will also depend on human actions (Jonas, 2013), hence the need for human agency. Containment of infectious diseases that spread between humans requires changes in human behaviours to disrupt the infection cycle. The Association for Professionals in Infection Control and Epidemiology (APIC) emphasize that "no matter the germ, there are six points at which the chain can be broken and a germ can be stopped from infecting another person" and these links are the infectious agent (the pathogen that causes the diseases); reservoir (places in the environment where the pathogen lives, e.g. humans, animals, insects); the portal of exit (the way the infectious agent leaves the reservoir, e.g. through aerosols, open wounds, a splatter of body fluids through coughing, sneezing); mode of transmission (the way the infectious agent is passed through direct or indirect contact, inhalation); a portal of entry (the way the infectious agent can enter the new host); and susceptible host (any vulnerable person) (APIC, 2016). Human action is necessary to break the chain of infection and risk communication plays a key role in influencing human behaviours required to break the spread of the disease. Advocacy and communication are key to behavioural changes required to disrupt the chain. Medical intervention alone will not break the chain. In a context like a coronavirus pandemic, where medical interventions like vaccines were not readily available, risk communication had a pivotal role in eliminating and reducing risk. As experiences from past pandemics show, individual and community responses depend on risk communications by authorities, private communications, public trust, public health measures, preparedness, and level of knowledge (Jonas, 2013). Failure in communications leads to the escalation of the crisis.

A pandemic is more than just a public health concern, as it has wide implications for all spheres of society. As evidenced from the past, most severe pandemics had a catastrophic impact on societies at large, inflicting huge human and economic losses. They had substantial negative impacts outside the health sector. In an article "The Price of Pandemics", Laura French writing for *World Finance* provides an overview of the economic effects brought by previous outbreaks like the Spanish Influenza, Zika, Swine Flu, and SARS. The financial estimates are staggering. Common to all these health crises is that the economic ramifications lasted for years. The International Monetary Fund forecast that the COVID-19 pandemic would cost the global economy USD 12.5 trillion by 2024 (Shalal, 2022). Public health crises are costly and potentially devastating to human life and society. The coronavirus pandemic is more than just a public health risk.

Emergency Risk and Crisis Communication

This book focuses on health risks, hence locating risk communication as essentially a type of crisis communication dealing with a public health concern. It also locates risk communication within the broader concept of health communication, a field that encompasses all forms of communication that seek to increase public awareness and educate the public about the nature of the disease – its causes, symptoms, and treatment. The public wants to know why, where, how, what about me, what should I do to avoid harm. Risk communication is critical to mitigate public health risk. Risk communication is used here to refer to "any public or private communication that informs individuals about the existence, nature, severity, or acceptability of risks" (Plough & Krimsky, 1987, p. 6). It means any "communication intended to supply laypeople with the information they need to make informed, independent judgements about risks to health, safety, and the environment" (Morgan, Fischhoff, Bostrom, & Atman, 2001). For WHO (2017), risk communication is an intervention to enable everyone to take informed decisions to protect themselves, their families, and communities against threats to their survival, health, and well-being.

Effective risk communication is communication that allows people most at risk to understand and adopt protective behaviours (WHO, 2017). This implies getting the right information to the right people at the right time, and above that, a certain degree of compliance to those messages. Risk communication covers a range of activities whose objectives are to provide the public with most of the answers they seek about the threat and most importantly, what they should do to physically protect themselves. When public safety is concerned, the public need information about how they can protect themselves from the ensuing danger, hence the need for Crisis and Emergency Risk Communication (CERC) (Ndlela, 2019). Risk communication is key to the containment of disease outbreaks and the prevention of other associated crises generated by the original crisis.

The overall risk and crisis communication during the coronavirus pandemic spanned a number of areas, including risk information, public health advice (mandated and recommendation), pandemic orders and rules, statistical information updates, and vaccination options and policies.

The term emergency risk communication is used here to denote a specific kind of communication used during emergencies such as public health crisis that evolve fast and need speedy intervention to eliminate or reduce the risk. The Centers for Disease Control's (CDC's) CERC describes "emergency" as "any public health event or incident presenting risk to life, health, and infrastructure including natural, weather-related, and manmade destruction, infectious disease outbreaks, and exposure to harmful biological, radiological, and chemical agents" (CDC, 2018). In a public health emergency like epidemics and pandemics, people's lives are at risk and they need urgent information that can aid risk avoidance. Barbara Reynolds, a senior crisis and risk communication advisor at CDC, emphasizes the importance of emergency risk communication thus: "the right message at the right time from the right person can save lives" (CDC, 2018). Relevant and accurate messages communicated timely from a trustworthy source can avert the impending crisis and save lives. A right message empowers decision-making among the stakeholders. The adage "the best way to manage a crisis is to prevent one" becomes even more relevant as the public needs to know what health risks they face and how they can protect their health and lives (Coombs, 2019).

In a pandemic emergency, there is no better way of managing the crisis other than slowing or breaking the rate of the infections through among other measures high risk awareness. The phrase "flatten the curve" gained traction in the beginning of the coronavirus pandemic as public health authorities raced to contain the virus by curbing the rate of infection to a level that could be accommodated by the healthcare system. If more people got infected with COVID-19 at the same time, the health infrastructure would collapse, further endangering the lives of other healthcare seekers. Such a situation would lead to other health crises. This created an emergency scenario that required risk messages and other measures that sought to help slow and reduce the infections. These measures called for a sustained risk communication effort to increase risk awareness. In risk situations like disease outbreaks, the quality, speed, and delivery of information are vital. As Freimuth et al. (2000) aptly put it: "increased emphasis on prevention have expanded the role of communication as a vital component of public health practice" (p. 337). Conversely, a low risk awareness would be like a mismanagement of a pandemic risk.

The Purpose of Risk Communication

Risk communication is an important component of public health emergency management. The main purpose of an emergence risk communication is to make the public understand the nature of the risk and the consequences that the risk poses to them as individuals, groups, organizations, or society. The general purpose of risk communication is to help manage the risk. This can involve attempts to eliminate the risk, mitigate its impact, or accept to live with it. Risk communication entails provision of information that individuals can use to make informed decisions about the risk and the choices they have. It also entails messages that seek to alleviate fear and anxiety. CERC ascribes the function of risk communication to providing the community with the information about the specific type (good or bad) and magnitude (strong or weak) of an outcome from an exposure

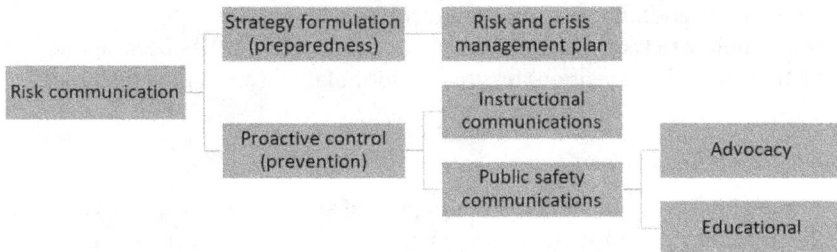

Figure 1.1 The purposes of risk communication.

or behaviour (CDC, 2018). Risk communication is identified by WHO as a core capacity of the International Health Regulations (IHR, 2005) and one of five strategies within the Pandemic Influenza Preparedness (PIP) framework:

> The purpose of risk communication is to enable people at risk to make informed decisions to mitigate the effects of a threat (hazard) – such as a disease outbreak – and take protective and preventive measures.
>
> (WHO, n.a)

The Institute of Medicine (1997) identified three purposes of risk communication: (a) advocacy, (b) education, and (c) promotion of decision-making. In relation to public health, advocacy has been conceptualized broadly to denote actions and processes that aim to strengthen the capacity of citizens to act on their own behalf to improve their health (Carlisle, 2000; Cohen & Marshall, 2017). It refers to all communication strategies and activities that seek to influence the target groups to change their behaviour in relation to a risk. Educational campaigns in public health crisis aim at giving people enough information about the risk so that they have enough knowledge to make their own decisions effectively. This includes edutainment approaches that use entertainment to attract the attention of target audiences. Given that the source of behaviour change or health behaviour is the individual (Piotrow & Kincaid, 2001), the goal of risk communication is to enable or promote decision-making and decision-making partnership by involving people actively in risk management options. The objectives are mutually interlinked.

Covello et al. (1987) distinguish four areas in which risk communication is applied: (1) informing and education, where people are informed and educated about the risks; (2) stimulating behavioural change and taking protective measures, which try to encourage risk reduction behaviour by influencing the perception of the audience; (3) disaster warnings and emergency information, which provide instructions and guidance during disasters and emergencies; and (4) exchange of information and a common approach to risk issues, which involve the public in risk management processes. Different types of risk will require different forms of risk communication. Figure 1.1 illustrates the different purposes of risk communication in public health emergencies.

In the field of crisis management, risk communication has been applied for proactive control (prevention) or strategy formulation (crisis preparedness).

Public Health Preparedness

Public health threats such as COVID-19 present significant global risks that need to be handled through national, regional, and global public policy and emergence management levels. When emerging public health risks are identified, assessed, and analysed, they have to be communicated to appropriate entities so that organizations at all levels can use the information to plan and take actions to mitigate the risks. The fact that a potential threat to public health was identified early is irrelevant if it is not communicated timely and effective to other global stakeholders, so that they also can plan and devise means to break the chain of infection. If a virus is allowed to spread, it will ultimately threaten everyone, hence the need for enhanced risk communication as a key preparedness ingredient. Accurate and timely risk communication in the event of an outbreak, epidemic, or pandemic enables public health authorities to devise appropriate risk and crisis management plans to help guide national and global responses to health emergencies. Improving global preparedness requires a clear understanding of threats to public health through effective risk communications and an understanding of how each state should respond, whether internally over its citizens or in co-operation with multinational organizations. In the context of public health emergencies, risk communication informs global health preparedness and crisis management planning. Emergency risk communication is a critical component of an effective response to public health emergencies (Seeger et al., 2018).

Instructional Communication

Proactive risk communication is the cornerstone of virtually every pandemic risk and crisis management. Even the most comprehensive pandemic response strategies will fail if they are not backed by sound risk communication. Proactive risk communication, as the name suggests, is a forward-thinking approach that focuses on identifying, analysing, and anticipating emerging risks and communicating them with the public for the purposes of preventive control. The main thrust is to avoid the emerging risk (or even eliminate it). Prevention strategies include, for example, public safety communications and warnings to the public. It can be warnings to inform the public about hazards, dangers, and risks in their environment. Such warnings include instructional communication as to how to deal with or avoid the hazards. The goal of such communication is to avoid or minimize the consequences of the hazards. It seeks to eliminate situations or events that, if they occur, can lead to injury or loss of property.

Coombs (2023) argues that people are the first priority in any crisis, and therefore organizations facing crisis should first and foremost instruct the public on how to avoid harm. Instructing information prioritizes the public's safety. Instructing information consists of all the messages sent during a crisis telling the people what to do to protect themselves physically from the crisis. In a crisis or emergency, people need to know what to do, for example, how to evacuate an area, find adequate shelter-in-place, boil drinking water, go somewhere for assistance, or return a defective product (Sturges, 1994). Coombs (2023) further argues that the instructing information reflects the desired response in a crisis. Sellnow and Sellnow (2010) argue that in order to protect the public in a crisis that increases health concerns, the communicators should apply the "instructional dynamic of risk communication". For example, during a food recall crisis, the communicators' primary concern is to instruct the public on which foods to avoid and how to either return or dispose of the dangerous product (ibid.). In emergencies, authorities need to provide instructional risk and crisis messages for self-protection and these messages ought to be clearly expressed and carefully selected (Sellnow & Sellnow, 2010). Instructional messages need to be delivered timely, as delays increase the risk of exposure to harm. On the contrary, lack of well-timed instructing information can lead to physical harm.

Crisis communication researchers, Sellnow and Sellnow (2011) conceptualized the IDEA model for effective instructional and crisis messages. The model, which is grounded in experimental learning theory, argues that learning is achieved when receivers not only understand information but also retain it accurately and use it appropriately. The model posits that effective instructional crisis messages ought to include four elements of a learning cycle model: Internalization (I), Distribution (D), Explanation (E), and Action (A). According to Sellnow and Sellnow (2011, 2013), internalization focuses on gaining and maintaining audience attention by demonstrating the relevance of the potential risk to them. They argue that explanations about the risk should be brief and understandable by the target audiences and should propose specific and meaningful actions that need to be taken. Finally, the messages should be distributed through those channels that are most likely to reach the target audiences. Sellnow et al. (2015) further argue that instructional risk and crisis messages that incorporate the IDEA framework are most likely to result in accurate and positive learning, hence achieve desired behavioural intentions.

Literature on risk and crisis communication concludes that instructional communication is an important aspect of the risk communication process and that effective instructional messages can motivate people to take appropriate protective action during a crisis (Edwards et al., 2021; Johansson, Lane, Sellnow, & Sellnow, 2021). Senders should communicate in a responsible and timely manner that clearly instructs the public what to do during a crisis event (Coombs, 2009; Covello, 1992; Sellnow et al., 2015). Instructional communication should have personal relevance, actionable directives, and adequate explanation (Sellnow et al., 2015).

While much of the literature has focused on top-down, sender-focused approaches, other researchers have emphasized the need for sender-focused approaches (Ndlela, 2019; Sellnow et al., 2015). Sender-focused approaches enable communicators to tailor the messages to specific audiences. Individual differences among receivers have a bearing on the reception of risk and crisis communication messages. Using demographic and psychographic segmentation can help identify traits within the audience. One of the challenges in complex risks and crisis is how to provide receivers with relevant information. Message tailoring is pivotal in any crisis communication.

Persuasive Communication

Persuasive risk communication is often used when the intention of the communicator is to change behaviour. It entails persuasive efforts by risk communicators to change the behaviours, attitudes, and opinions of specific groups or stakeholders regarding a risk issue. Miller (1980) defines persuasive communication as any message that is intended to shape, reinforce, or change the responses of another or others. Persuasion includes "any effort to modify an individual's evaluation of people, objects or issues by the presentation of a message" (Petty & Cacioppo, 1987, p. 25). Persuasive communication emphasizes the notion of change, be it change of attitude, behaviour, habits, emotions, or beliefs about a risk or issue. Hence, any message that is intended to shape, reinforce, or change the responses of another or others will be defined as persuasive communication (Stiff, 1994, p. 10).

Several strands of research from different disciplines such as behavioural science, psychology, and political science exist in message effect studies. The message effect research of the 1960s attempted to define the characteristics of persuasive messages. In his book *Persuasive Communication*, James Stiff describes some of the prominent strands in message effect studies:

Rational persuasion: "Persuasive messages that contain rational arguments based on the assumption that people have an implicit understanding of formal rules of logic, and that they apply these rules when making judgements about a source's recommendation" (Stiff, 1994, p. 108). The emphasis of communication is placed on the quality of evidence that is offered to support the conclusion. Rational persuasion emphasizes the importance of supporting information. However, the persuasiveness of the message is dependent on the motivation and ability of the recipient to process the message contained in the message (Petty & Cacioppo, 1987). People who are motivated and fully engaged with the risk issue are more likely to fully scrutinize the message than those who are less engaged. Different people engage differently in risk issues and hence the importance of adapting the message to their degree of engagement. Their degree of engagement and their ability to interpret the message is a determinant factor in the understanding of the message and the attitude to change. As such, rational persuasion techniques require that the targeted people make an active effort in receiving and processing the risk message.

Emotional persuasive appeal: In many persuasive contexts, the message recipients are unable or unmotivated to effectively process rational appeals, and hence, under these circumstances, persuaders often turn to emotional persuasive appeals (Stiff, 1994). Emotional appeals tap into the subconscious as opposed to the conscious mind. This approach uses the manipulation of emotions to influence message recipients. This approach is used in different fields, including marketing and advertising, where communicators target the subconscious mind through eye-catching adverts. Fear appeals have been used in prevention and safety campaigns, such as Don't Drink and Drive campaigns, the use of seat belts, cigarette smoking, and HIV/AIDS. In these campaigns, fear-arousing messages, often accompanied by gruesome images, have been used to motivate the target groups to change their behaviour or attitude. The aim is to make an emotional appeal to the people to change their behaviour and attitude towards a potential risk.

Effective Risk and Crisis Communication

Crisis communication experts have for decades endeavoured to describe "best practices" in crisis communication and risk communication as a way of improving professional practice. Literature on risk and crisis communication identifies predominant elements that constitute the basis for effective communication. The seminal work of Cutlip and Center (1952) identified 7Cs that form the basis of good communication, that is, to be clear, concise, concrete, correct, coherent, complete, and courteous. Covello (2003) provides nine checklists of best practices that should be included in any public health risk and crisis plan. Seeger (2006) and Heath (2006) articulate a set of best practices for crisis and risk communication. Seeger cautions that "the best practices are general standards rather than specific prescriptions about methods, channels, and messages" (p. 242). Led by the CDC, scholars, including Belinda Reynolds and Matthew Seeger, have attempted to merge traditional notions of health and risk communication with work in crisis and disaster communication into a more comprehensive approach called the CERC Model (Reynolds & Seeger, 2005). The six principles in the CDC's CERC manual are:

1 *Be First*: Crises are time-sensitive. Communicating information quickly is crucial. For members of the public, the first source of information often becomes the preferred source.
2 *Be Right*: Accuracy establishes credibility. Information can include what is known, what is not known, and what is being done to fill in the gaps.
3 *Be Credible*: Honesty and truthfulness should not be compromised during crises.
4 *Express Empathy*: Crises create harm and the suffering should be acknowledged in words. Addressing what people are feeling and the challenges they face build trust and rapport.
5 *Promote Action*: Giving people meaningful things to do calms anxiety, helps restore order, and promotes some sense of control.
6 *Show Respect*: Respectful communication is particularly important when people feel vulnerable. Respectful communication promotes co-operation and rapport (CDC, 2018).

Examples and discussions in the next chapters would highlight some of the successes and challenges in relation to these ideal principles.

Conclusion

This chapter has presented the context for the book, which focuses more broadly on risk and crisis communication and more particularly on the challenges to effective communication messages, responses to the pandemic, and the lessons learned from COVID-19 pandemic. Since its outbreak, the coronavirus has disrupted everyday life, virtually affecting every sphere of life, be it work, education, business, religions, relationships, and cultural activities. It became imperative for governments around the world to inform their citizens about the impending health risk and the ongoing pandemic. Communication is the essence of any crisis and disaster management. Pandemics affect people and communication is the sine qua non of human existence and survival. As the WHO correctly notes: "It is the people who matter most, and without the people we have no disaster" (WHO, 2002).[1] Yet, communication about the COVID-19 to the audiences encountered several challenges due to various factors, some of which are examined in this book. The pandemic took place in an entirely transformed digital communication landscape, which provides both opportunities and disadvantages for crisis communication. The following chapters in this book provide insights into the challenges associated with communicating COVID-19 messages.

Note

1 https://lms.must.ac.ug/claroline/backends/download.php?url=Lzc2NTZfd2hhd
   F9pc19kaXNhc3Rlci5wZGY%3D&cidReset=true&cidReq=BALFP3209_001
   (Accessed 20.06.2023).

References

APIC. (2016). Break the Chain of Infection, Infection prevention and you. *Association for Professionals in Infection Control and Epidemiology*. https://infectionprevention-andyou.org/protect-your-patients/break-the-chain-of-infection/ (Accessed 20.06.2023)

Beck, U. (2009). *World of Risks* (C. Cronin, Trans.). Cambridge: Polity Press.

Bicchieri, C., Fatas, E., Aldama, A., Casas, A., Deshpande, I., Lauro, M., . . . Wen, R. (2021). In science we (should) trust: Expectations and compliance across nine countries during the COVID-19 pandemic. *PLoS One*, *16*(6), e0252892. doi:10.1371/journal.pone.0252892

Boin, A., 't Hart, P., Stern, E., & Sundelius, B. (2016). *The Politics of Crisis Management: Public Leadership under Pressure* (2 ed.). Cambridge: Cambridge University Press.

Carlisle, S. (2000). Health promotion, advocacy and health inequalities: A conceptual framework. *Health Promotion International, 15*(4), 369–376. doi:10.1093/heapro/15.4.369

CDC. (2018). Crisis and emergency risk communication. Center for preparedness and response (CPR) Retrieved from https://emergency.cdc.gov/cerc/manual/index.asp

Cohen, B. E., & Marshall, S. G. (2017). Does public health advocacy seek to redress health inequities? *A Scoping Review, 25*(2), 309–328. doi:10.1111/hsc.12320

Coombs, W. T. (2009). Conceptualizing crisis communication. In R. L. Heath & H. D. O`Hair (Eds.), *Handbook of Crisis and Risk Communication* (pp. 100–119). New York: Routledge.

Coombs, W. T. (2019). *Ongoing Crisis Communication. Planning, Managing, and Responding* (5 ed.). Los Angeles, CA: Sage.

Coombs, W. T. (2023). *Ongoing Crisis Communication. Planning, Managing, and Responding* (6 ed.). Thousand Oaks, CA: Sage.

Covello, V. T. (1992). Trust and credibility in risk communication. *Health and Environment Digest, 6*(1), 1–4.

Covello, V. T. (2003). Best practices in public health risk and crisis communication. *Journal of Health Communication, 8*(1), 5–8. doi:10.1080/713851971

Covello, V. T., Winterfeldt, D., & Slovic, P. (Eds.). (1987). *Uncertainty in Risk Assessment, Risk Management, and Decision Making.* New York: Plenum Press.

Cutlip, S. M., & Center, A. H. (1952). *Effective Public Relations: Pathways to Public Favor.* New York: Prentice-Hall.

Edwards, A. L., Sellnow, T. L., Sellnow, D. D., Iverson, J., Parrish, A., & Dritz, S. (2021). Communities of practice as purveyors of instructional communication during crises. *Communication Education, 70*(1), 49–70. doi:10.1080/03634523.2020.1802053

Freimuth, V., Linnan, H., W., & Potter, P. (2000). Communicating the threat of emerging infections to the public. *Emerging Infectious Diseases, 6*(4), 337–347.

French, L. (2022, 31.01.2023). *The Price of Pandemics.* London: World Finance. https://www.worldfinance.com/strategy/the-price-of-pandemics (Accessed 20.06.2023)

Heath, R. L. (2006). Best Practices in crisis communication: Evolution of practice through research. *Journal of Applied Communication Research, 34*(3), 245–248. doi:10.1080/00909880600771577

Institute of Medicine. (1997). Risk communication and vaccination: Workshop summary (9780309573627). Retrieved from Washington, US: https://pubmed.ncbi.nlm.nih.gov/25121223/

Johansson, B., Ihlen, Ø., Lindholm, J., & Blach-Ørsten, M. (2023). *Communicating a Pandemic: Crisis Management and Covid-19 in the Nordic Countries.* Gothenberg: Nordicom.

Johansson, B., Lane, D. R., Sellnow, D., D., & Sellnow, T. L. (2021). No heat, no electricity, no water, oh no!: an IDEA model experiment in instructional risk communication. *Journal of Risk Research, 24*(12), 1576–1588. doi:10.1080/13669877.2021.1894468

Johnsson, B., Solhberg, J., & Esaiasson, P. (2023). Institutional trust and crisis management in high-trust societies. In B. Johansson, Ø. Ihlen, J. Lindholm, & M. Blach-Ørsten (Eds.), *Communicating a Pandemic: Crisis Management and Covid-19 in the Nordic Countries* (pp. 285–302). Gothenburg: Nordicom.

Jonas, O. (2013). Pandemic risk. https://openknowledge.worldbank.org/bitstream/handle/10986/16343/WDR14_bp_Pandemic_Risk_Jonas.pdf?sequence=1&isAllowed=y

Lerbinger, O. (1997). *The Crisis Manager: Facing Risk and Responsibility.* New Jersey: Lawrence Erlbaum.

Levitt, A. M. (1997). *Disaster Planning and Recovery: A Guide for Facility Professionals.* New York: John Wiley & Sons.

Miller, G. R. (1980). On being persuaded: Some basic distinctions. In G. R. Miller & M. E. Roloff (Eds.), *Persuasion: New Directions in Theory and Research* (pp. 16–17). Beverly Hills, CA: Sage Publications.

Morgan, M. G., Fischhoff, B., Bostrom, A., & Atman, C. J. (2001). *Risk Communication: A Mental Models Approach.* New York: Cambridge University Press.

Ndlela, M. (2019). *Crisis Communication: A Stakeholder Perspective.* Cham, Switzerland: Palgrave Macmillan.

Ndlela, M. (2021). The coronavirus pandemic in Africa: Crisis communication challenges. *Journal of African Media Studies, 13*(2), 133–138. doi:10.1386/jams_00039_2

Petty, R. E., & Cacioppo, J. T. (1987). *Communication and Persuasion: Central and Peripheral Routes to Attitude Change.* New York: Springer-Verlag.

Piotrow, P. T., & Kincaid, D. L. (2001). Strategic communication for international health programs. In R. Rice & C. Atkin (Eds.), *Public Communication Campaigns* (pp. 249–266). Third Edition, Thousand Oaks, CA: Sage Publications.

Plough, A., & Krimsky, S. (1987). The emergence of risk communication studies: Social and political context. *Science, Technology & Human Values, 12*(3&4), 4–10.

Pond, P. (2020). *Complexity, Digital Media and Post Truth Politics. A theory of Interactive Systems.* Cham, Switzerland: Palgrave Macmillan.

Reuters. (2020). Wuhan lockdown 'unprecedented', shows commitment to contain virus: WHO representative in China. https://www.reuters.com/article/us-china-health-who-idUSKBN1ZM1G9

Reynolds, B., & Seeger, M. W. (2005). Crisis and emergency risk communication as an integrative model. *Journal of Health Communication, 10*(1), 43–55.

Santini, R. M., Salles, D., Tucci, G., Ferreira, F., & Grael, F. (2020). Making up audience: Media bots and the falsification of the public sphere. *Communication Studies, 71*(3), 466–487. doi:10.1080/10510974.2020.1735466

Seeger, M. W. (2006). Best practices in crisis communication: An expert panel process. *Journal of Applied Communication Research, 34*(3), 232–244. doi:10.1080/00909880600769944

Seeger, M. W., Pechta, L. E., Price, S. M., Lubell, K. M., Rose, D. A., Sapru, S., . . . Smith, B. J. (2018). A conceptual model for evaluating emergency risk communication in public health. *Health Security, 16*(3), 193–203. doi:10.1089/hs.2018.0020

Sellnow, D. D., Lane, D., Littlefield, R. S., Sellnow, T. L., Wilson, B., Beauchamp, K., & Venette, S. (2015). A receiver-based approach to effective instructional crisis communication. *Journal of Contingencies and Crisis Management, 23*(3), 149–158. doi:10.1111/1468-5973.12066

Sellnow, D. D., Lane, D. R., Sellnow, T. L., & Littlefield, R. S. (2017). The IDEA model as a best practice for effective instructional risk and crisis communication. *Communication Studies, 68*(5), 552–567. doi:10.1080/10510974.2017.1375535

Sellnow, T. L., & Seeger, M. W. (2021). *Theorizing Crisis Communication* (2 ed.). Hoboken, NJ: Wiley-Blackwell.

Sellnow, T. L., & Sellnow, D. D. (2010). The instructional dynamic of risk and crisis communication: distinguishing instructional messages from dialogue. *Review of Communication*, 10(2), 112–126. doi:10.1080/15358590903402200

Sellnow, T. L., & Sellnow, D. D. (2011). *Messages Matter: Crisis Communication Strategies for Encouraging Self-Protection*. Little Rock, AR: Center for Toxicology and Environmental Health.

Sellnow, T. L., & Sellnow, D. D. (2013). The role of instructional risk messages in communicating about food safety. *Food Insight: Current Topics in Food Safety Nutrition*. International Food Information Council Foundation.

Shalal, A. (2022). IMF sees cost of COVID pandemic rising beyond $12.5 trillion estimate. https://www.reuters.com/business/imf-sees-cost-covid-pandemic-rising-beyond-125-trillion-estimate-2022-01-20/

Sinatra, G. M., & Hofer, B. K. (2021). *Science Denial. Why It Happens and What to Do about It*. Oxford: Oxford University Press.

Stiff, J. B. (1994). *Persuasive Communication*. New York: The Guilford Press.

Sturges, D. L. (1994). Communicating through crisis. *Management Communication Quarterly*, 7(3), 297–316. doi:10.1177/0893318994007003004

Sulik, J., Deroy, O., Dezecache, G., Newson, M., Zhao, Y., El Zein, M., & Tunçgenç, B. (2021). Facing the pandemic with trust in science. *Humanities and Social Sciences Communications*, 8(1), 301. doi:10.1057/s41599-021-00982-9

WHO. (2002). Disasters and emergencies. Definitions. Training package, Panafrican Emergency Training Centre, Addis Ababa, WHO/ AHA https://lms.must.ac.ug/claroline/backends/download.php?url=Lzc2NTZfd2hhdF9pc19kaXNhc3Rlci5wZGY%3D&cidReset=true&cidReq=BALFP3209_001 (Accessed 20.06.2023).

WHO. (2017). Communicating risk in public health emergencies: A WHO guideline for emergency risk communication (ERC) policy and practice. https://apps.who.int/iris/bitstream/handle/10665/259807/9789241550208-eng.pdf

WHO. (2020). WHO Director-General's opening remarks at the media briefing on COVID-19-11 March 2020, https://www.who.int/director-general/speeches/detail/who-director-general-s-opening-remarks-at-the-media-briefing-on-covid-19---11-march-2020 (Accessed 20.06.2023).

WHO. (n.a). Risk communications and community engagement (RCCE). https://www.who.int/emergencies/risk-communications

2 COVID-19

An Unexpected Pandemic?

Introduction

The coronavirus pandemic has been peddled as one of those rare events, the unforeseen, unexpected crises. In simple terms, rare events are seldom events that occur with low frequency and that have widespread impact. Lampel et al. (2009) provide two perspectives on rare events. The first perspective defines rare events as "probability estimates, usually calculated from the frequency of the event". In this perspective, collected data inform decisions on whether an event is rare or not. Defining the event as rare affect preparedness thinking as organizations are most likely to invest more time and efforts in the prevention of those events that are most likely to occur and less in those that are least likely to occur. The probability perspective defines rare events from quantitative measures. The second perspective defines rare events "as opportunities for unique sensemaking based on the enacted salience of specific features of the rare events" (Lampel et al., 2009, p. 835).

Lampel et al. (2009) argue that there are "no rare events" as such because these can only be defined in a particular context. Events are more likely to be considered rare if individuals or organizations that experience or observe these events see them as unusual. Hence, events are only rare relative to specific decision-makers, or put in another way, the same event can be rare for one organization but commonplace for another. This is transferrable to disease outbreaks that can be rare in certain territories but common occurrences in others. The coronavirus 2019 (COVID-19) pandemic has exposed the deficit of pandemic preparedness by decision-makers. COVID-19 is a rare event that has proven to be less improbable than thought. Since pandemics are rare, there was a significant lack of preparation for the coronavirus pandemic. In their article "Lack of preparation for rare events", Maćkowiak and Wiederholt (2018) note the following: "a rare event occurs, agents who did not prepare for the rare event because it was unlikely take bad actions, and catastrophic consequences follow". The catastrophic consequences are a direct result of the lack of preparedness. They further argue that since the incentives to prepare for a rare event are small, few

DOI: 10.4324/9781003401827-2

agents will be prepared when the rare event occurs (Bartosz & Mirko, 2020). The COVID-19 pandemic shares these features as prominent world leaders and public health authorities have openly admitted that the world was not prepared for this kind of pandemic. Little guidance as to how to act in a rare event has implications for crisis management and risk communication messages.

The Pandemic – The Black Swan or the Gray Rhino?

The COVID-19 pandemic, sweeping around the world like wildfire since December 2019, appeared to be very much rare, leading some to variously characterize it as a *Black Swan* event or a *Gray Rhino* event. The two metaphors drawn from the works of Nassim Taleb and Michele Wucker have been used to characterize large-scale crises. The Black Swan is a metaphor coined by Nassim Taleb in his book *The Black Swan: The Impact of the Highly Improbable* (2007). It draws on the widely held belief that a black swan did not exist. The belief persisted among the people until a black swan was seen in Australia. Black swans are not as rare as previously thought. Taleb describes a black swan as a *highly improbable* event that is *unpredictable* and carries a massive impact. It describes any event that "seems to us, based on our limited experience, to be impossible" (Taleb, 2007). Some people have described the COVID-19 pandemic as a black swan. Undoubtedly, describing the event as a black swan absolves authorities and decision-makers who do not need to be accountable for their failures to prepare for the eventuality. In a comment in *The New Yorker* (2020), Taleb noted that a black swan has become a "cliché for any bad thing that surprises us".

Unlike the improbable and unpredictable black swans, a Gray Rhino event "is a highly probable, high impact threat: something we ought to see coming" (Wucker, 2016, p. 7). Wucker uses the metaphor of the Elephant in the Room to show that Gray Rhino is something we ought to be able to see by the virtue of its size. Yet, to the contrary, we fail to recognize the obvious. These are "threats that we ought to see but often don't see, or that we see but wilfully ignore" (p. 15). Gray Rhinos are predictable well in advance; they give multiple warnings that they could happen and hence can be avoided or minimized if correct preventive measures are taken. Writing on pandemics, Wucker (2016) notes that "the frequency of pandemics warns of a much bigger global health threat to come: it's not a matter of *if*, but *when*" (p. 7).

Was the pandemic unforeseen? A cursory look at some national risk reports shows that public health authorities were fully aware of the possibilities of a disease outbreak or even a pandemic that could have serious consequences for life, health, and the economy. For example, yearly reports by the Norwegian Institute of Public Health, dating back as far as 2013,[1] have repeatedly noted that vulnerabilities for diseases that are easily transmitted through droplet infection or airborne infection, to which few or none are naturally immune and where there is no existing vaccination or treatment, are high in all societies. The reports state explicitly that "no society can efficiently shut out such diseases" because travel connection between countries and continents increases the likelihood of infectious diseases. How serious the consequences will be depend on the characteristics of the virus and *society's ability to deal with the pandemic*, both in terms of reducing the spread of infection, treating the sick, and handling it in general.

A TED talk by Bill Gates in March 2015, "The next outbreak? We're not ready", pointed out that the greatest risk of global catastrophe was the outbreak of a virus rather than a war. He bemoaned that the world was not ready and had invested very little in systems to stop an epidemic. That a pandemic was likely to happen was not a question of "if" but "when". The threat of a global disease was something the world leaders could have seen. As Wucker argues, "the biggest threat facing leaders are not highly improbable Black Swans, but highly probable Gray Rhinos. We may not be able to foresee the details or the timing, but the outlines of the biggest threats facing us are hard to ignore" (p. 15). The above illustrates that the threat of a global disease outbreak was probable and foreseeable.

Yet to world authorities, there was no way to predict that an outbreak in China would escalate into a pandemic. There have been numerous outbreaks before and most of these fizzled out. As the World Health Organization (WHO) aptly put it: we have never before seen a pandemic sparked by a coronavirus. This is the first pandemic caused by a coronavirus." Similarly, the then US President Donald Trump, expressed that "nobody knew there'd be a pandemic or an epidemic of this proportion. Nobody's ever seen anything like this before.[2]

Pandemics in History

Outbreaks are fraught with surprises that can unsettle even the most developed preparedness plans. Yet, human history is awash with outbreak stories where epidemics and pandemics brought much human suffering and caused many fatalities. Since time immemorial, different parts of the world have experienced many outbreaks, epidemics, and pandemics. These three concepts distinguish the level and intensity of the disease. Turner (2020) provides a distinction between these concepts using the metaphor of a ladder. At the bottom of an epidemiological ladder is an outbreak, defined in *The Merriam-Webster* dictionary as "a sudden rise in the incidence of a disease".[3] Disease outbreaks occur frequently. Between 1 May 2002 and 31 March 2005, the WHO detected 760 outbreaks with a potential for international concern and in 2020, 74 outbreaks were registered and these include SARS-Cov-2 variants, yellow fever, Ebola, Avian Influenza A (H5N1), MERS-CoV, and many more (Wilder-Smith & Osman 2020). Although outbreaks are nearly constant, few of these reach epidemic or pandemic levels, that is, stages higher in the epidemiological ladder. In the middle of the ladder is an epidemic – "an outbreak of contagious disease that has become more severe and less localized".[4] WHO (2018) registered a total of 1,307 epidemic events globally between 2011 and 2017. What distinguishes epidemics and pandemics is the prevalence of the infectious disease. At the top of the ladder is a pandemic, defined as a global outbreak of a contagious disease (Turner, 2020).

More than a dozen pandemics have been experienced throughout history. Since 1500, more than 18 pandemics have been registered, with interval periods ranging from 10 to 40 years. In a review article "History of the Plague: An Ancient Pandemic for the Age of COVID-19", Glatter and Finkelman (2021) provide a succinct overview of the plague epidemics that have afflicted humanity for thousands of years. Early pandemics include the Black Death or Bubonic plague which killed more than 25 million people or a third of the European population between 1347 and 1352. The plague spread across most of Europe leaving a swath of agony on its path. Those who contracted the disease died within a week of contracting it. Outbreaks of the plague broke out now and then across Europe for the next 400 years. Bramanti et al. (2016) describe the Bubonic plague as a pandemic which changed the path of human civilization due to demographic, social, and economic consequences in Western European countries.

Another plague pandemic broke out in southwestern China around 1855 and spread globally via maritime shipping (Bramanti et al., 2016; Glatter & Finkelman, 2021). The pandemic affected Asia, America, and Africa. The pandemic took millions of lives, with more than 2.2 million in China alone, and an estimated 12 million people died from the plague in India between 1898 and 1918 (Perry & Fetherston, 1997).

In the past century alone, pandemic influenza viruses have emerged three times, that is, the 1918 "Spanish" Influenza (H1N1), the 1957 "Asian Influenza", (H2N2) and the "Hong Kong" Influenza (H3N2) (Schwartz & Kapila, 2021). The Spanish flu, also known as the 1918 H1N1 killed an estimated 20–50 million people worldwide (Tumpey et al., 2005). The Asian flu of 1957 originated in northern China and spread into neighbouring countries, before spreading around the world. It is estimated that about 1.1 million died worldwide.

In late 2002, there was an outbreak of severe acute respiratory syndrome (SARS) in the Guangdong Province in China. Despite efforts by the Chinese government and WHO to contain the transmission, SARS spread to "5 countries within 24 hours and to more than 30 countries on 6 continents within 6 months" (Schmiege et al., 2020). SARS quickly spread along the routes of international air travel. Similarly, a novel influenza A (HINI) virus was detected in the USA in 2009, and by 2010, it had spread to over 214 countries. In June 2011, WHO declared A (H1N1) a pandemic.

Another outbreak which caused a global scare was the Ebola virus epidemic, recorded first in Guinea in 2013 before spreading widely to the neighbouring countries of Sierra Leone and Liberia, with smaller outbreaks in Nigeria, Mali, and Senegal, and with imported cases registered in the USA, Spain, the UK, and

Norway. The Ebola epidemic caused fear and panic around the world, but it did not escalate into a pandemic. The crisis exposed fissures in the global health response and deficiencies in public health communication.

The coronavirus pandemic is just one in an already long list of public health crises. The pandemic should therefore be understood within the historical context of epidemics and pandemics. Platto et al. (2021) note in their research that the SARS-CoV-2 virus of the COVID-19 pandemic had been active well before January 2020, when its pathogenic potential exploded full force in Wuhan, China. Smaller outbreaks of the disease had been occurring in China and elsewhere in the world, without necessarily becoming epidemic. Unexpectedly, the outbreak in the late 2019s came with increased transmissibility and hence the globalization of the infection. Since then, the coronavirus has spread throughout the world like wildfire, infecting millions of people in more than 223 countries. By February 2021, confirmed cases of infection reached over 106 million, with more than two million deaths. In an age of global interconnectedness, the probability of further continued transmission to other parts of the world was very high. Increased connectivity, especially in air and rail travel, increased the possibilities of human contact. Even though China tried to isolate the outbreak area by taking unprecedented actions, such as suspending all public transportation, lockdown of Wuhan and other cities in Hubei, and restricting the movement of millions of people in the province, it did not prevent the virus from reaching distant shores. Increased global mobility propelled transmission into Europe and the USA and continued to spread to other parts of the world.

Public Health Preparedness

Researchers in crisis management emphasize a proactive approach to preparing for unforeseen events, be it the Black Swans or Gray Rhinos. They emphasize that situational awareness is imperative as new threats can emerge anytime and anywhere. The risk of a pandemic spread is more present than ever before. Factors such as global travel, climate change, and animal-human contact are likely to fuel infectious diseases and other unforeseen events. Unforeseen events are types of uncertainty conditions that disrupt the normal course of time (Lampel et al., 2009). These events test the adaptability of an organization's current intentions, rules, routines, and regulations to new situations, often uncovering blind spots and weaknesses in functionality (Netz, Svensson, & Brundin, 2020; Roux-Dufort, 2007). Epidemics and pandemics in the past decades gave public health authorities the world over a better understanding of the complexities and dynamics of a global spread. Experiences from previous outbreaks show that the world is not immune to epidemics and pandemics; hence the need for preparedness and prevention (also known as mitigation). Many strides have been achieved in bolstering preparedness and many potential pandemic diseases have been contained. Outbreaks like Ebola exposed fissures in the global preparedness for public health emergencies. The experience of the Ebola outbreak emphasized the need to increase disease surveillance, response measures, and develop robust health information systems.

The concept of "preparedness" is common in the different areas of crisis management, with various prefixes such as *disaster preparedness, emergency preparedness*, and *public health preparedness*. Preparedness is invariably used to categorize actions that pre-emptively enhance the response to a disaster (Sellers, Crilly, & Ranse, 2022). Concerning public health, the WHO describes disaster preparedness as having multiple components, including identifying potential hazards, developing a stockpile of available resources, and establishing the capacity to respond to a health emergency (Sellers et al., 2022). Pandemic preparedness involves meaningful practices for detection, response, and recovery to disease outbreaks from local to global levels.

However, preparedness remains a rather broad and ambiguous concept, imprecise as to what is needed to achieve the state of preparedness. As Coccia (2022) argues, one of the fundamental problems is the measurement of the preparedness of countries to cope with the pandemic threats. While it remains unclear what the exact driving factors of better preparedness are, there is a general agreement on the need for countries to be prepared to reduce the negative impact of the pandemic in terms of mortality and in preventing the spread. Noting the failures in the coronavirus pandemic, the Global Preparedness Monitoring Board (GPMB) published a report aptly titled "From Worlds Apart to a World Prepared" (GPMB, 2021). The report argues that the failures in the COVID-19 response were rooted in inequality and inaction.

Preparedness is a vital aspect of proactive crisis management and communication. Being proactive entails taking several measures to prevent or mitigate the crisis. All necessary steps should be taken to avoid a crisis in the first place. Crisis prevention is a proactive approach to crisis management, where the impetus is geared towards stopping a crisis event from happening. The adages "the best way to manage a crisis is to prevent one" (Coombs, 2019) and "the second best way to manage a crisis is to prepare for one" (Frandsen & Johansen, 2017) point to the implied significance of crisis prevention and crisis preparedness. If a crisis does not happen, no one is harmed. Timothy W. Coombs argues however that prevention is a rather strong word since not all crises can be prevented. He prefers the term *mitigation*. Mitigation means to lessen the effects of something (Coombs, 2019). From a health crisis perspective, prevention is the most widely used. In health epidemics and pandemics like COVID-19, the primary goal is both *preventing* the transmission and *mitigating* the impact. In this book, the concepts are placed on a continuum – preparedness, prevention-mitigation, and response and recovery.

Prevention and mitigation are crucial measures in the containment of epidemics and pandemics. The world is chronically vulnerable to many infectious diseases, some of which are known while others are unknown. Most of these cannot be fully prevented, but public health authorities can only hope to mitigate their effects. Authorities take actions designed to eliminate the crisis threat or to reduce the likelihood of the threat becoming a crisis. Hence, one way of mitigating the impact of the pandemic is to protect the health system and ensure continuity of services during and after the pandemic. As the WHO notes, "when an epidemic emerges and spreads, it inevitably draws most of health responders' attention and monopolizes most of the health system's human and financial resources, as well as medical products and technologies" (WHO, 2018). Epidemics and pandemics divert attention from everyday health services, resulting in the neglect of basic and essential health services. They put national health systems under great pressure and stress. The unintended consequence is the increase in mortality rates of other diseases.

Crisis mitigation during an epidemic and pandemic is about preserving the health system by slowing down the rate of disease transmission. Maintaining a state of equilibrium is essential to preserve the capacity and resources of national health systems. A grim scenario during the COVID-19 pandemic was the possibility of the number of COVID-19 patients needing respirators surpassing the intensive care capacity. Hence, as the number of cases of COVID-19 outside China increased and the number of affected countries tripled, WHO expressed concern about not only the levels of spread and severity of COVID-19 but also "the alarming levels of inaction". As the number of infected people increased exponentially, the coronavirus erupted into a full-on pandemic. Mathematical models predicted huge numbers of infections and hospitalization. There were fears across the world that the continued ascent in the curves will soon surpass national health capacities and culminate in a disaster. The curves all pointed towards a dire situation, where the number of people gasping for oxygen in the intensive care units exceeded the available resources in hospitals. The COVID-19 pandemic sent shockwaves throughout the world, as panic-stricken public health authorities set into action their response plans, unaware that some poor countries hardly had any prepared plans.

The Pandemic Crisis Response

When the WHO declared the novel coronavirus a pandemic, governments had to engage the public health crisis. In any crisis, as Coombs (2023) points out, all crisis actions have to be communicated to the stakeholders, both internal and external, who could be affected by the actions. Critical in any crisis response and central to the crisis *response* stage is the strategic deployment of different forms of communications. Crisis responding centres on the risk and crisis communication messages are created and sent to different stakeholders and target groups. These messages are informed by the crisis strategy options as well as the tactical considerations. The strategic aspects of the pandemic message pertain to the goals and objectives of the communicating organization. Crisis communication is a form of strategic communication due to its goal orientation (Coombs, 2023). Since crises in general disrupt the pursuit of organizational goals, crisis communication creates temporary goals required to navigate this disruption to strategy (Coombs & Holladay, 2022). The strategic focus of crisis communication looks at what the messages seek to achieve. During a pandemic, the overall strategic goal is to increase awareness of the risk and promote risk-averting behaviours. The pandemic response messages seek to protect public safety and ensure physical safety and psychological well-being. It is the objectives that guide the strategy. The tactical consideration in the pandemic response pertains to the form of the crisis response, that is, the speed of the response, the consistency of the messages, and the issues of openness in the communication. Prevention and preparedness are key foundations for responsive crisis communication. Carefully planned crisis communication messages are pivotal to the prevention and mitigation of public health threats.

Conclusion

While the coronavirus caught public health authorities by surprise and has been touted as a rare unforeseen and unexpected event, there are indications that a pandemic was highly probable. There were several signals that such as public health threat was eminent, and the question was not *if* but *when*, as aptly put by Wucker (2016). Yet, when the pandemic came, public authorities were not ready for the outbreak. A pandemic is much more that a public health crisis. It is a mega-crisis with ramifications across every sector. The response to the crisis ignites a myriad of other crises such as socio-economic and psychological crises (the pandemic impacts the mental health of many people, increasing levels of fear, stress, anxiety, depression, frustration, and uncertainty). Managing pandemics involve more than just medical interventions. Where vaccines or medicines are not readily available, the only plausible alternative is to give the public information about the risk and what they should do to prevent harm to themselves. The lack of preparedness for the COVID-19 pandemic had a negative bearing on risk crisis communication messages. The coronavirus pandemic has been characterized by varying degrees of muddled messages from political leadership, public health authorities, and scientific experts.

Notes

1 Utbrudd av smittsomme sykdommer i Norge. Årsrapport 2013. Utgitt av Nasjonalt folkehelseinstitutt, Divisjon for smittevern. Juli 2014 www.fhi.no (quoted in https://www.dsb.no/globalassets/dokumenter/rapporter/nrb_2014.pdf)
2 https://www.npr.org/transcripts/827692672 (Accessed 10.05.2022).
3 https://www.merriam-webster.com/dictionary/epidemic (Accessed 11.02.21).
4 https://www.merriam-webster.com/dictionary/epidemic (Accessed 11.02.21).

References

Bartosz, M., & Mirko, W. (2020). Lack of preparation for rare events and policy implications in the time of COVID-19. https://voxeu.org/article/lack-preparation-rare-events-and-policy-implications-time-covid-19

Bramanti, B., Stenseth, N.C., Walløe, L., & X, L. (2016). Plague: A disease which changed the path of human civilization. In R. Yang & A. A. (Eds.), *Yersinia Pestis: Retrospective and Perspective. Advances in Experimental Medicine and Biology, vol 918* (pp. 1–26). Dordrecht: Springer.

Coccia, M. (2022). Preparedness of countries to face COVID-19 pandemic crisis: Strategic positioning and factors supporting effective strategies of prevention of pandemic threats. *Environmental Research, 203*, 111678. doi:10.1016/j.envres.2021.111678

Coombs, W. T. (2019). *Ongoing Crisis Communication: Planning, Managing, and Responding* (5 ed.). Los Angeles, CA: Sage.

Coombs, W. T. (2023). *Ongoing Crisis Communication: Planning, Managing, and Responding* (6 ed.). Thousand Oaks, CA: Sage.

Coombs, W. T., & Holladay, S. (2022). Crisis communication as strategic communication: Process and insights. In J. Falkheimer & M. Heide (Eds.), *Research Handbook on Strategic Communication* (pp. 259–273). Cheltenham: Edward Elgar Publishing.

Frandsen, F., & Johansen, W. (2017). *Organizational Crisis Communication*. Los Angeles: Sage.

Glatter, K. A., & Finkelman, P. (2021). History of the plague: An ancient pandemic for the age of COVID-19. *The American Journal of Medicine, 134*(2), 176–181. doi:10.1016/j.amjmed.2020.08.019

GPMB. (2021). From worlds apart to a world prepared. Retrieved from https://www.gpmb.org/docs/librariesprovider17/default-document-library/gpmb-annual-report-2021.pdf?sfvrsn=44d10dfa_9

Lampel, J., Shamsie, J., & Shapira, Z. (2009). Experiencing the improbable: Rare events and organizational learning. *Organization Science, 20*(5), 835–845. doi:10.1287/orsc.1090.0479

Maćkowiak, B., & Wiederholt, M. (2018). Lack of preparation for rare events. *Journal of Monetary Economics, 100*, 35–47. doi:10.1016/j.jmoneco.2018.07.007

Netz, J., Svensson, M., & Brundin, E. (2020). Business disruptions and affective reactions: A strategy-as-practice perspective on fast strategic decision making. *Long Range Planning, 53*(5), 101910. doi:10.1016/j.lrp.2019.101910

Perry, R. D., & Fetherston, J. D. (1997). Yersinia pestis - Etiologic agent of plague. *Clinical Microbiology Reviews, 10*(1), 35–66. doi:10.1128/cmr.10.1.35

Platto, S., Wang, Y., Zhou, J., & Carafoli, E. (2021). History of the COVID-19 pandemic: Origin, explosion, worldwide spreading. *Biochemical and Biophysical Research Communications. 538*, 14–23. doi:10.1016/j.bbrc.2020.10.087

Roux-Dufort, C. (2007). Is crisis management (only) a management of exceptions? *Journal of Contingencies and Crisis Management, 15*(2), 105–114. doi:10.1111/j.1468-5973.2007.00507.x

Schmiege, D., Perez Arredondo, A. M., Ntajal, J., Minetto Gellert Paris, J., Savi, M. K., Patel, K., . . . Falkenberg, T. (2020). One Health in the context of coronavirus outbreaks: A systematic literature review. *One Health, 10*, 100170. doi:10.1016/j.onehlt.2020.100170

Schwartz, R. A., & Kapila, R. (2021). Pandemics throughout the centuries. *Clinics in Dermatology.* 39(1), 5–8. doi:10.1016/j.clindermatol.2020.12.006

Sellers, D., Crilly, J., & Ranse, J. (2022). Disaster preparedness: A concept analysis and its application to the intensive care unit. *Australian Critical Care.* 35(2), 204–209. doi:10.1016/j.aucc.2021.04.005

Tumpey, T. M., Basler, C. F., Aguilar, P. V., Zeng, H., Solórzano, A., Swayne, D. E., . . . García-Sastre, A. (2005). Characterization of the reconstructed 1918 Spanish influenza pandemic virus. *Science, 310*(5745), 77–80. doi:10.1126/science.1119392

Turner, J. A. (2020). Pandemics and epidemics through history: This too shall pass. *Journal of Hospital Librarianship, 20*(3), 280–287. doi:10.1080/15323269.2020.1779540

WHO. (2018). Managing epidemics: Key facts about major deadly diseases [Press release].

Wilder-Smith, A., & Osman, S. (2020). Public health emergencies of international concern: a historic overview. *Journal of Travel Medicine,* 27(8), taaa227. https://doi.org/10.1093/jtm/taaa227

Wucker, M. (2016). *The Gray Rhino: How to Recognize and Act on the Obvious Dangers We Ignore.* New York: St. Martin's Press.

3 The World's First Digital Pandemic

Introduction

Developments in new information and communication technologies continue to shape and reshape the communication landscape for risk and crisis communication messages. The new communication environment brings to the fore new affordances, limitations, and challenges for crisis management. Issues of audience fragmentation, the declining role of gatekeepers, and the increasing influence of algorithms, bots, and autonomous agents in the digital communication sphere, in a different way influence the communication process. These changes invariably change ways of communicating with target audiences during public health emergencies. The infrastructure of communication technology is more complex today than it was in the previous public health crisis. One of the noticeable developments relates to the increased datafication of communication and society. Algorithmic data processes and autonomous tools are significantly changing the foundations of communication, including risk and crisis communication. Due to huge amounts of data generated, analysed, and consumed during the pandemic, some researchers have proclaimed that this is the first "data-driven pandemic" (Shelton, 2020). The coronavirus pandemic is unique, in that it is the first pandemic to occur in an era of widespread digital communication, more particularly "mobile-device-supported social media, Big Data and AI" (Gaffield, 2021). The concept of digital communication is often used to cover a broad area of communications, mostly the technical aspects of the digital transmission of information. Developments in digital communications have revolutionized the way organizations communicate and interact with their public. They are changing the interfaces between crisis communicators and their audiences. It is an incontrovertible fact that we are now in the midst of revolutionary changes in the sphere of digital communications, characterized by extensive connections via mobile devices. Social media platforms seamlessly connect people, defying the confines of place, space, and time. Information flows in digital spaces to the recipients (pc, mobile, tablet) within a fraction of a second.

DOI: 10.4324/9781003401827-3

Informational technologies, more particularly social media and mobile telephony, have wrought fundamental changes to crisis communication. The new technologies have fundamentally altered the processes of production, distribution, and consumption of information during a crisis. Social media has evolved since its inception into a complex and potent force of communication during crises. Digital communication facilitated communication during the pandemic and has undoubtedly played an important role in the efforts to combat the coronavirus. Davis and Matsoso (2020) aptly capture this assertion in their article published in the *Think Global Health* newsletter:

> Covid-19 was a moment of global digital transformation. From the moment the disease was identified, every potential and pitfall of our data arsenal rose to the surface, from artificial intelligence (AI) algorithms promising to speed us toward new vaccine candidates, to powerful surveillance and visualization tools helping to map the disease's trajectory, to the head-spinning power of social media apps connecting the dots within communities – as well as being vehicles for both spreading and combatting misinformation

Unlike in any pandemic before, authorities resorted to digital instruments for a wide array of services, be it information, surveillance, tracking, monitoring, or management of data. The public alike turned to digital communication platforms for messages and other communication needs. Networks of scientists collaborated on their research, thanks to digital collaborative platforms. Similarly, journalists around the world have been able to collaborate on their stories. Besides these positive attributes of digital communication, we witnessed another set of challenges that arguably set dampers on crisis communication efforts. The following characteristics of digital communication have a profound impact on communication messages during a crisis.

Audience Fragmentation

Digitalization opens a diversity of communication platforms and tools that can be harnessed for crisis communication purposes. It incorporates real-time communication capabilities such as voice, video, and messaging in their interaction with their stakeholders. Channel digitalization has expanded the number of channels for crisis communication. Unlike in the past, when citizens gathered around a few broadcasting stations or print media for news about the crisis, today people with access to the internet have an infinite number of digital media channels, including numerous social media platforms. These are easily accessible via the now ubiquitous mobile telephones. The internet and social network platforms, weblogs, microblogging, podcasts, wikis, content communities, and many others have transformed the production, distribution, and consumption of crisis news. In some countries, internet and the social media is now the preferred medium of everyday communication. In the USA, for example, according to the Pew Research Center, more than eight-in-ten adults say that they get their news from a smartphone, computer, or tablet often, whether it is a news website or search and social media (Shearer, 2021). These include news websites run by non-mainstream media institutions and other sources that claim to be news organizations. News sites saw a surge in popularity mainly due to polarization in society on COVID-19 pandemic issues. In Scandinavian countries, research shows a higher level of trust in media institutions which became central to COVID-19 messages (Diaz et al., 2020; Johnsson, Ihlen, Lindholm, & Blach-Ørsten, 2023). Nevertheless, these countries have segments of the population such as immigrant communities and the youth that do not rely on the mainstream media for sources of COVID-19 messages.

In the past, crisis communicators had fewer communication channels to consider and use to convey important messages to the public. The new digital media landscape brings to the fore new opportunities, but also enormous challenges for crisis communicators. It is undoubtedly easy and cheaper to communicate, but the communication landscape is now complex and audiences are fragmented (Fletcher & Nielsen, 2017). Some audiences are not easy to reach in these fragmented contexts. Communicators have to tailor their messages to numerous channels, from word-limited platforms like Twitter to video-based platforms. There is no guarantee that messages will ever reach the intended audiences simply because they have been published. It is no longer easy to attract public attention to vital information due to a constant flow of content, including algorithm-driven content (Kaluža, 2022; Napoli, 2019). With channel plurality comes also the dangers of false information, propaganda, and other content that flourishes in digital media and floods out pandemic messages (Adeitan, Onyechi, & Omah, 2021; Dwoskin, 2021; UNICEF, 2021). If we contrast the current situation and the past, we notice some glaring differences. For example, during the Ebola epidemic in West Africa in 2016, the penetration of the internet and mobile telephone was relatively low in those regions and the challenge then was the lack of modern communication tools to reach the public with public health messages (Nyenswah, Engineer, & Peters, 2016; Ratzan & Moritsugu, 2014). Fast forward to 2020, the dynamics had changed and the challenge now has been how to combat misinformation circulating on popular social media platforms like WhatsApp.

Algorithms, Bots, and AI

Recent advances in communication and human-machine communication are transforming all the facets of crisis communication messages (Beer, 2017; Bucher, 2017; DeVito, 2017; Ferrara, Varol, Davis, Menczer, & Flammini, 2016). Technologies such as automatic text generators, social media bots, and voice assistants present new opportunities and challenges for crisis communication.

They perform the role of communicator and moderator in the communication process. In the social media era, there is a growing influence of non-human communicators like algorithms and bots in news and information production, dissemination, and consumption (Howard, Woolley, & Calo, 2018). These computational means are used to inflate stories, amplify them through bots, create fake following in social media, and generally distort the flow of information during a crisis. "Bots are software intended to perform simple, repetitive, robotic tasks such as delivering news and information, whether real or junk – or undertake malicious activities like spamming, harassment and hate speech" (Neudert, Kollany, & Howard, 2017). Bots mimic and potentially manipulate humans and their behaviours on social networks. They run automatically to produce messages, post online, and interact with users through likes, comments, and follows (fake accounts). Bots in social media platforms can disseminate messages, replicate themselves, and even cause people to believe that they are human users, thereby manipulating public opinion (Dahir, 2018; Natale, 2021; Ndlela, 2020).

Algorithms determine the flow of information on social media networks. Huge amount of data are produced in social media platforms. Algorithms help handle these huge amounts of information by, among other functions, sorting, filtering, and dispensing information into an individual's story feeds based on a predetermined set of criteria such as the type of content, amount of activity around the content, and connection between users. Algorithms watch user-digital behaviours, the devices they use, the websites they visit, and all the content they interact with social media platforms or the internet and then make assumptions and predictions on user preferences. Based on these predictions, they filter and recommend similar content to the user. In so doing, algorithms determine the visibility and invisibility of content, meaning that a user is more likely to be exposed to the content from those closest to him/her or based on his/her digital behaviour. The result of this selective exposure is the creation of some form of filter bubbles (Kaluža, 2021; Koc-Michalska, 2017; Makhortykh & Wijermars, 2021). This phenomenon is at the heart of filter bubble studies, which have looked at the implication of algorithms and the ultimate creation of knowledge centres or epistemic bubbles. Classic examples include the polarized knowledge centres (epistemic bubbles) around specific issues, for example, climate change. During the coronavirus pandemic, we saw the rise of epistemic bubbles around the pro- and anti-vaccination groups. Users in these groups were most likely to receive algorithmic-driven feeds that reinforced their position.

Automated dissemination of large volumes of misinformation, fake news, and sensational news over social networks of family and friends has impacted the types of knowledge available to the public. Automated accounts and dissemination algorithms influence the content and traffic online. Social media flourishes with machine-generated information, including manipulated, deceptive, and incorrect information, existing alongside correct and relevant information, thus complicating knowledge formation processes. Natale (2021) aptly refers to these technologies based on artificial intelligence (AI) as deceitful media, due to their ability to project agency and humanity, as she argues: "deception is a constitutive element of AI rather than an unwelcome by-product" (p. 1). The element of deception is central to the functioning of AI. For an audience that is already overwhelmed with information these machine-generated messages not only increase information floods that drown useful messages but deceive the audience. People inundated with information might find it difficult to distinguish between correct and false, useful and un-useful information, thereby infringing on their ability to understand the risks associated with the coronavirus, make sense of the prevailing crisis, or take correct decisions to protect themselves.

Manipulable Messages

Another distinguishable characteristic of the digital age is that everything in media content is manipulable. The availability of cheaper or free editing software means that an average person can edit text, voice, and pictures in any content. With voice editing software, original voice can be manipulated, replaced, or completely removed quickly and then deceptively passed on to other users as being authentic. A worrisome development is the rise of deepfakes, the use of a form of AI called deep learning, to digitally alter videos and replace the person or voice in the original video with someone else's in a way that makes the content look authentic. Until recently, it was difficult to alter video content, but today, just about anyone with the right software can create a convincing fake video. Some of the deepfakes videos exploit the images of trusted or prominent persons, either for fun memes or even to promote certain agendas. One can recall the deepfakes featuring former US presidents Barack Obama and Donald Trump. The darker side of deepfakes is that during a crisis, they have been used to convey false or misleading information and promote agendas that undermine crisis response messages. Deepfakes manipulate speeches for the sake of a misinformation campaign, distort discourses, erode trust, damage reputations, and jeopardize public safety. Fact-checking agencies have struggled to keep pace with the scourge of sophisticated deepfakes that have become increasingly difficult to detect.

The same applies to text and picture editing tools, which enable the changing of original content. During the pandemic, this editing software has been used for various purposes, ranging from creating humorous memes to impersonation of public authorities. Users have circulated information purporting to be government statements. For example, in Zimbabwe, a purported statement regarding an extension of the national lockdown was circulated early in April 2020. The statement carried the president's signature, looked authentic, and was meant to deceive the readers (Aljazeera, 2020). False messages undoubtedly create confusion and undermine crisis response messages.

False information using letterheads of reputable organizations and falsified statistical information are some examples concerning the vulnerability of messages in the digital communication environment. Other documents vulnerable to falsification were COVID-19 test certificates adopted to allow uninfected people to travel internationally or enter local arrangements and restaurants. Fake certificates proliferated as the black market for fake COVID-19 vaccines and certificates emerged to take advantage of the situation. Many countries, including the UK, Dubai, Zimbabwe, Mozambique, South Africa, and South and Central America, encountered falsified or fake certificates (Hausenkamph, 2021). Even the EU's digital certificate with a QR code and digital signature was susceptible to fraud. As Hausenkamph notes, in France, real certificates with real QR codes were being sold in the black market. In Namibia, two men operating a printing shop were arrested for printing fake COVID-19 negative results for truck drivers who needed them to cross into neighbouring countries. These examples illustrate how any digitalized information can be changed and passed on as "real". Falsification of information undermines efforts to convey useful messages that contribute positively to tackling the threats of infectious disease. The obvious implication for crisis management is that we live in an era where messages can easily be manipulated to create other sets of information and meanings.

Active Audiences

Another characteristic of the digital era is that of active audiences. Digital communication has removed all communication barriers, creating interchangeable roles for producers and consumers. People are no longer passive recipients, targets, empty vessels waiting to be filled with messages (Jaffe & Jaffe, 2007). In the social media context, communicators no longer control the reach of their messages, the audiences do. Exposure to a message in a social media context is also a by-product of viewers who voluntarily rate and rank content, sharing it with friend networks or re-posted it on content-sharing sites. The sharing capabilities afforded in social media can make messages, both original and falsified, reach distant places. Communicators have lost control of their content and the reach, frequency, and timing of the distribution of their messages. The audience can hijack crisis messages and turn them into jokes or parodies for entertainment purposes, thus stripping them of their seriousness. Another aspect of social media is that content drives audience interaction in social media. In today's competitive digital world, crisis communicators are under pressure to produce enough content to gratify audience demands before they lose interest and go on to other content providers. Gaining the attention of the audience has become difficult.

The Decline of Gatekeepers

Digital communication has brought new challenges to crisis and risk communication messages. Before the advent of digital communication and social media, society relied on the mass media (radio, television, and newspapers) and periodicals for crisis information. The news media were the most important source of information during major crises. Everything the public read or saw was filtered through by journalists, editors, and other news production staff. The principles of the "old" media were based on a "one-to-many" communication process, whereby communication went from one sender to multiple receivers through a medium such as a radio, newspaper, magazine, or television. In this process, only a few (e.g. journalists) wrote messages that were then disseminated to many recipients through the mass media. In times of crisis, authorities could address the nation directly through radio or television. Message recipients had limited opportunity, if any, to respond to messages.

Important in the past was the role of gatekeepers – the mass media – in ensuring that only certain crisis messages formulated in certain ways were transmitted to the receivers. Gatekeeping involves a series of processes for deciding which messages reach audiences. Gatekeeping is defined as "the process by which the vast array of potential news messages is winnowed, shaped, and prodded into those few that are transmitted by the news media" (Shoemaker, Eichholz, Kim, & Wringley, 2001). Gatekeepers facilitate or constrain the diffusion of information as they decide which messages to allow past the gates (Shoemaker & Vos, 2009). Through filtering processes, gatekeepers ensured that "billions of messages that are available in the world get cut down and transformed into the hundreds of messages that reach a given person on a given day" (p. 3).

The classical gatekeeping theory provides a solid framework for how the media filtered information reaching society (Vos & Russell, 2019). Since its inception, the mass media have served as gatekeepers to what information reaches society and how that information was framed. Gatekeeping involves more than just gatekeeping; it includes decisions such as the selection of information, framing, display, the timing of publication as well as withholding or repeating certain aspects of the message. The traditional mass media, or what has been described as the fourth estate, derives its power to hold other institutions accountable to the public power through its gatekeeping. This power entails many things, including the selection and prioritization of news items, deciding the sources of information that can be used in the stories, editing, and ensuring the quality of information and dissemination of information. The media had full control and responsibility for the content.

The media gatekeepers have been very crucial in times of crisis, selecting news, framing, and reporting about the crisis. The power of the media extended to controlling the sources of information and deciding which voices could be heard by society. During crises, this power becomes eminent as the media set boundaries on who was allowed and not allowed into the public sphere. Hence, only certain voices (institutions and individuals) got access to the media while other voices were marginalized. Media news affects the formation of public opinion.

In this communication context, public authorities needed to devise strategies for using or influencing the news media, which were considered to be a crucial interface between authorities and the public. It meant that they put a lot of strategic effort into the construction of news content through media relations strategies (Jonkman, Trilling, Verhoeven, & Vliegenthart, 2019). Literature shows that "transmitting messages to the public through mass media, arranging positive news coverage and communicating with journalists on organizational issues have always been situated at the heart of public relations" (Verhoeven, 2016). Press releases have been an instrumental source of information for journalists.

In gatekeeping, process information is filtered through many stages before reaching the receivers, who very often have little or no opportunities for responding to the messages. Public communication is based on one-to-many logic and emphasize a one-way information flow. This gives the sender gatekeeping control in information dissemination. In a one-to-many model, communication flows in one direction from one centre to many target groups. A few in societies, for example, in the organization's communication department or media house, decide and select the type of content to be shared with the intended target groups. Often guided by certain goals and objectives, they decide the message to be read, heard, or seen by others as well as the medium to be used. The medium can be a letter, telephone, newsletter, or any communication via the mass media. Even though the sender retained much control of information, the mass media were the ultimate gatekeepers regulating access to the wider society. For example, even if an organization issued a news release, the decision to publish it or not and what was finally communicated to the readers or viewers rested with the editors or publishers. Not every press release got published. Other messages also depended on the few publishers – those who owned both the production and distribution means.

New Forms of Gatekeeping

The rise of the internet saw organizations turning to the internet for communications through websites and other information portals. The internet provided opportunities for organizations to provide first-hand information to whoever had access to the internet and had an interest in the organization. The internet gave organizations the possibility to reach their constituencies directly without going through intermediaries such as the mass media. The organization's website also served as the immediate source of information for journalists. Based on the results of a content analysis of the websites of Fortune 500 companies, Callison (2003) notes how corporate websites became the journalists' first choice of information when a story broke and no live source was available. As the percentage of journalists using the internet for article research increased, PR practitioners realized the power internet afforded them in enhancing media relations. The internet gave access to the growth of online newspapers or newspaper-like publications that are neither owned by traditional media institutions nor manned by trained journalists.

The internet is however not free from gatekeepers. The concept of "online gatekeeper" has been used in discussing gatekeeping implications of search engines, news portals, and algorithms in the digital arena (Evans, Jackson, & Murphy, 2022; Kruse, 2011). Hargittai (2000) argues that gatekeeping activity still occurs online, but now takes place at the level of information exposure. It determines what consumers hear and know about. In a blog article "The Internet's Gatekeepers?", Kruse (2011) argues that "as long as there has been information, there have been gatekeepers who control it". The communication practitioners are also gatekeepers to information about the organization. For example, intranet editors are the main corporate gatekeepers and agenda setters making news publication decisions, that is, determining what is important and newsworthy (Lehmuskallio, 2008). Very often, they seek to protect the organization's identity and reputation, influence public opinion, and generally shield the organization from negative exposure. Like journalists, information practitioners decide what is newsworthy as well as how to frame "bad news".

Wang and Zhu (2019) use the concept of collective gatekeeping to refer to information aggregation services provided by social news websites (SNWs), where users' collaborative information filtering such as voting, comments, and recommendations are effective drivers for news diffusion. Through SNWs such as Digg, Reddit, Delicious, and Newsvine, users can submit, share, and comment on the news. Even though SNWs are technically based on social networking services (SNS), they are more concerned with information sharing, unlike friendship-centred social media like Facebook. Users are hence also crucial to the diffusion of information. As Wang and Zhu (2019) argue, "SNW fosters online citizen journalism and underlines the transformation of news diffusion from mass communication to a participatory process" (p. 36). They further assert that when an individual user decides whether to share information or not, they act as a gatekeeper to control the information flow in their local community (network). Sharing of news potentially increases chances for more sharing. Social media allows the new audience to communicate with each other and with other gatekeepers. The role of gatekeeping is exchangeable in the social media context.

In the era of digital communication, it is however difficult to fully control messages due to the multitude of senders and receivers. In the internet sphere, communications and interactions are also initiated by non-human elements. Automated communication systems send information and recommend news, products, and services to receivers based on their user profiles or digital footprints. Based on digital profiles and tracking of internet uses, automatic machines send users recommendations on news, services, and products they assume are of interest. Automated communications are part of the new world of crisis communications. Crisis communication is now enmeshed in a complex and multidimensional process involving one-to-one, one-to-many, and many-to-many communications, one-to-community communication, multiple communities, and networked communities. Interactivity is also the main characteristic of this new communication environment.

Many-to-Many Communication

Digital communication technology supports many-to-many communication flow, in which messages flow from many sources to many receivers. Anybody can easily become a content producer, publisher, or consumer at the same time. Users are interconnected and information flows in seamless directions. Many-to-many communication is characterized by "No start. No end. No sender. No receiver. Just fluidity. Continuity" (Jaffe & Jaffe, 2007, p. 16). In social media, the sender and receiver roles are interchangeable. Roles shift with today's sender becoming tomorrow's receiver. In the many-to-many model, there is no dominant player, but there are initiators. Anyone with something to say can initiate and drive the communication. Examples include mass mailing (email), retweets, and sharing in social media that allow the users to disseminate information to one or millions of other users at the same time. This form of communication is a threat to the control of risk and crisis messages. It distributes power and transcends geographical boundaries. Many-to-many communication allows what Pfister (2011) refers to as a new model of "participatory expertise" which challenges traditional routines of knowledge production, disrupts information routines, and cultivates multi-perspectivalism. A good example is the emergent forms of "networked expertise" such as Wikipedia, which allow for "information flows from multiple, often peripheral, nodal points toward a central, aggregating node" (Pfister, 2011, p. 218). Digital communication technologies can "sustain large-scale, interlinked, synchronous and asynchronous contacts" and hence lead to even more complex societies.

Many-to-many communication represents a more fundamental shift in the processes of knowledge production and dissemination during crises. Digital communication technology expands the "who contributes to subject matter expertise from the one to many" (Pfister, 2011, p. 222). In a digital world, knowledge production itself is dispersed and epistemic authority is continuously challenged by other "experts", "non-experts", online commentators, bloggers, influencers, anarchists, and conspiracy theorists. In modern society, experts and their authority are no longer unquestioned. For example, as Bruckman (2004) argues, many-to-many communication is changing the nature of medicine as new medical consumers are better informed. Research by the Pew Center for Internet Life in the USA shows that many adult Americans have used the internet to access health and medical information. Patients talk with other individuals with similar conditions and exchange information and knowledge on many digital platforms. Modern patients face their doctors armed with printouts from WebMD, other internet-based diagnostics, and other medical information sourced through social media.

Many-to-many communication had a profound influence on crisis and risk communication messages during a pandemic. During the pandemic, digital communication facilitated the networking of scientists around the world working on different aspects of COVID-19-related research. It also facilitated the emergence of other sources of scientific knowledge that either concurred with or opposed existing knowledge about the coronavirus. People sought not only official centres of epistemic authority but also other available knowledge sources, in addition to creating their knowledge. As such, during the pandemic, we witnessed the emergency and visibility of multiple centres of knowledge, which vied for attention in the rhetorical arenas. Some of these centres constituted themselves into closed virtual communities of like-minded thinkers where they circulate only messages that amplified or reinforced their ideas. This situation creates echo chambers and filter bubbles where a person only encounters information or opinions that reflect or reinforce their own (Nguyen, 2020). Those inside the bubble are not exposed to other messages, resulting in fragmented societies. Even though the digital communication environment allows for multiperspectival information, some people are exposed to single perspectives. For example, anti-vaccinationists, sometimes referred to as "anti-vaxxers" or "antivax", are most likely to be exposed to information that reinforces their views against vaccination received from other members of the anti-vax communities.

Another important characteristic of social media is its interactivity and speed. Social media allows users to share and exchange information, knowledge, and opinions rather quickly. These characteristics increase the information dispensation at a speed not envisaged before.

Influencers as Sources of News

Influencers are increasingly important in crisis news dissemination. Social media have seen a rise of new potent forces of one-to-many communicators with the power to influence many of their followers. It is no longer media institutions alone sending their products to the masses, but also some influential individuals with many followers. An influencer is someone who has built an audience, naturally and over time, and is viewed as an authority on a certain subject, area, or perspective in the online space (Freberg, 2019). Influencers have established credibility in a specific area, have access to a huge audience, and are trusted by their followers, something which allows the influencers to persuade their audiences to take specific action based on what is shared (ibid., p. 171). Influencers have a following on different social media platforms like Twitter, Instagram,

Facebook, YouTube, and Snapchat. The primary focus of the influencers is to drive conversations on issues of interest on social media platforms. Some influencers manage to tap over a million followers in one or across platforms. For example, Markplier, known for gaming videos and sketches, has over 30 million followers across platforms. On Twitter, we have individuals like the former US President Barack Obama (130 million), Kim Kardashian (70 million), India's Prime Minister Narendra Modi (72.4 million), Bill Gates (56 million), and former US President Donald Trump (88.9 million) with millions of followers. There are several national macro- and micro-influencers that potentially tilt the balance of scale in communicating COVID-19 messages. Individuals with many followers have the power to influence public opinions, perceptions, and behaviours. Their role during a crisis cannot be underestimated.

Conclusion

This chapter has provided a background to the digital communication environment that confronted the coronavirus risk and crisis communication messages. During a public health emergency, communicators deal with the challenges of selecting appropriate channels to deliver messages to increasingly fragmented audiences. Given the increased number of channels available for crisis communication and the fragmentation of the audiences, crisis communication has become a complex endeavour. The variety of channels available and their affordances, limitations, and challenges can be overwhelming to overstretched crisis communicators. Finding an audience in specialized and localized information outlets with varying characteristics can be daunting during an emergency. While it can be tempting to use as many channels as possible to reach the target audiences, co-ordinating the messages across platforms to ensure consistency can be another challenge. This chapter has also shown how algorithms increasingly affect the flow of crisis messages in digital communication platforms. The coronavirus pandemic fits the characterization of being the world's first digital pandemic.

References

Adeitan, M. A., Onyechi, N. J., & Omah, O. (2021). COVID-19 containment and control: Information source credibility and adoption of prevention strategies among residents in South West Nigeria. *Journal of African Media Studies, 13*(2), 235–251. doi:10.1386/jams_00046_1

Aljazeera. (2020). Zimbabwe president threatens fake news author with 20 years' jail. https://www.aljazeera.com/economy/2020/4/14/zimbabwe-president-threatens-fake-news-author-with-20-years-jail

Beer, D. (2017). The social power of algorithms. *Information, Communication & Society, 20*(1), 1–13. doi:10.1080/1369118X.2016.1216147

Bruckman, A. (2004). Many-to-many communication: A new medium. In National Research Council of the National Academies, *Computer Science: Reflections on the Field, Reflections from the Field* (pp. 134–143). Washington, DC.: The National Academies Press.

Bucher, T. (2017). The algorithmic imaginary: Exploring the ordinary affects of Facebook algorithms. *Information, Communication & Society, 20*(1), 30–44. doi:10.1080/1369118X.2016.1154086

Callison, C. (2003). Media relations and the Internet: how Fortune 500 company web sites assist journalists in news gathering. *Public Relations Review, 29*(1), 29–41. doi:10.1016/S0363-8111(02)00196-0

Dahir, A. L. (2018). How social media bots became an influential force in Africa's elections. https://qz.com/africa/1330494/twitter-bots-in-kenya-lesotho-senegal-equatorial-guinea-elections/

Davis, S., & Matsoso, P. (2020). COVID-19 as a digital pandemic. *Think Global Health.* July 7, 2020, https://www.thinkglobalhealth.org/article/covid-19-digital-pandemic (Accessed 20.06.2023).

DeVito, M. A. (2017). From editors to algorithms. *Digital Journalism, 5*(6), 753–773. doi:10.1080/21670811.2016.1178592

Diaz, E., Norredam, M., Aradhya, S., Benfield, T., Krasnik, A., Madar, A., & Juarez, S. (2020). Situational brief: Migration and Covid-19 in Scandinavian countries. https://migrationhealth.org/wp-content/uploads/2021/05/lancet-migration-situational-brief-skandinavia-01-en.pdf

Dwoskin, E. (2021). On social media, vaccine misinformation mixes with extreme faith. *The Washington Post.* Retrieved from https://www.washingtonpost.com/technology/2021/02/16/covid-vaccine-misinformation-evangelical-mark-beast/

Evans, R., Jackson, D., & Murphy, J. (2022). Google news and machine gatekeepers: algorithmic personalisation and news diversity in online news search. *Digital Journalism*, 1–19. doi:10.1080/21670811.2022.2055596

Ferrara, E., Varol, O., Davis, C., Menczer, F., & Flammini, A. (2016). The rise of social bots. *Communications of the Acm, 59* (7), 96–104. doi:10.1145/2818717

Fletcher, R., & Nielsen, R. K. (2017). Are news audiences increasingly fragmented? A cross-national comparative analysis of cross-platform news audience fragmentation and duplication. *Journal of Communication, 67*(4), 476–498. doi:10.1111/jcom.12315

Freberg, K. (2019). *Social Media for Strategic Communication.* Los Angeles: Sage.

Gaffield, C. (2021). The world's reaction to the first pandemic of the digital era. https://digitalfuturesociety.com/qanda/the-worlds-reaction-to-the-first-pandemic-of-the-digital-era-by-chad-gaffield/

Hargittai, E. (2000). The digital divide and what to do about it. In D. C. Jones (Ed.), *New Economy Handbook.* San Diego, CA: Academic Press.

Hausenkamph, D. S. (2021). Covid-19 Vaccine Certificates: The Digitalisation of Fraud.

Howard, P. N., Woolley, S., & Calo, R. (2018). Algorithms, bots, and political communication in the US 2016 election: The challenge of automated political communication for election law and administration. *Journal of Information Technology & Politics, 15*(2), 81–93. doi:10.1080/19331681.2018.1448735

Jaffe, J., & Jaffe, J. (2007). *Join the Conversation: How to Engage Marketing-Weary Consumers with the Power of Community, Dialogue, and Partnership.* Hoboken: John Wiley & Sons, Incorporated.

Johnsson, B., Ihlen, Ø., Lindholm, J., & Blach-Ørsten, M. (2023). Introduction: Communicating a pandemic in the Nordic countries. In B. Johnsson, Ø. Ihlen, J. LIndholm, & M. Blach-Ørsten (Eds.), *Communicating a Pandemic: Crisis Management and Covid-19 in the Nordic Countries* (pp. 11–30). Gothenburg, Sweden: Nordicom.

Jonkman, J. G. F., Trilling, D., Verhoeven, P., & Vliegenthart, R. (2019). To Pass or Not to Pass: How Corporate Characteristics Affect Corporate Visibility and Tone in Company News Coverage. *Journalism Studies, 21*(1) 1–18. doi:10.1080/14616 70X.2019.1612266

Kaluža, J. (2022). Habitual generation of filter bubbles: Why is algorithmic personalisation problematic for the democratic public sphere? *Javnost - The Public, 29*(3) 267–283. doi:10.1080/13183222.2021.2003052

Koc-Michalska, K. (2017). Helping populism win? Social media use, filter bubbles, and support for populist presidential candidates in the 2016 US election campaign AU - Groshek, Jacob. *Information, Communication & Society, 20*(9), 1389–1407. doi:10.10 80/1369118X.2017.1329334

Kruse, E. (2011). The internet's gatekeepers? Retrieved from https://www.ericsson.com/ en/blog/2011/8/the-internets-gatekeepers

Lehmuskallio, S. (2008). Intranet editors as corporate gatekeepers and agenda setters. *Corporate Communications: An International Journal, 13*(1), pp. 95–111.

Makhortykh, M., & Wijermars, M. (2021). Can filter bubbles protect information freedom? Discussions of algorithmic news recommenders in Eastern Europe. *Digital Journalism*, 1–25. doi:10.1080/21670811.2021.1970601

Napoli, P. (2019). Algorithmic gatekeeping and the transformation of news organizations. In P. Napoli (Ed.), *Social Media and the Public Interest* (pp. 53–79). New York: Columbia University Press.

Natale, S. (2021). *Deceitful Media: Artificial Intelligence and Social Life after the Turing Test*. New York: Oxford University Press.

Ndlela, M. (2020). Social media algorithms, bots and elections in Africa. In M. N. Ndlela & W. Mano (Eds.), *Social Media and Elections in Africa, Volume 1: Theoretical Perspectives and Election Campaigns* (pp. 13–37). Cham: Springer International Publishing.

Neudert, L.-M., Kollany, B., & Howard, P. (2017). Junk news and bots during the German parliamentary election: What are German voters sharing over Twitter? Oxford, UK. Retrieved from https://demtech.oii.ox.ac.uk/research/posts/junk-news-and-bots-during-the-german-parliamentary-election-what-are-german-voters-sharing-over-twitter/

Nguyen, C. T. (2020). Echo chamber and epistemic bubbles. *Episteme, 17*(2), 141–161. doi:10.1017/epi.2018.32

Nyenswah, T., Engineer, C. Y., & Peters, D. H. (2016). Leadership in times of crisis: The example of Ebola virus disease in Liberia. *Health Systems & Reform, 2*(3), 194–207. doi:10.1080/23288604.2016.1222793

Pfister, D. S. (2011). Networked expertise in the era of many-to-many communication: On Wikipedia and invention. *Social Epistemology, 25*(3), 217–231. doi:10.1080/0269 1728.2011.578306

Ratzan, S. C., & Moritsugu, K. P. (2014). Ebola crisis—communication chaos we can avoid. *Journal of Health Communication, 19*(11), 1213–1215. doi:10.1080/10810730. 2014.977680

Shearer, E. (2021). *More Than Eight-in-Ten Americans Get News from Digital Devices.* Pew Research Center. https://www.pewresearch.org/short-reads/2021/01/12/more-than-eight-in-ten-americans-get-news-from-digital-devices/ (Accessed 20.06.2023).

Shelton, T. (2020). A post-truth pandemic? *Big Data & Society, 7*(2), 2053951720965612. doi:10.1177/2053951720965612

Shoemaker, P. J., Eichholz, M., Kim, E., & Wringley, B. (2001). Individual and Routine Forces in Gatekeeping. *Journalism & Mass Communication Quarterly, 78*(2), 233–246.

Shoemaker, P. J., & Vos, T. P. (2009). *Gatekeeping Theory.* New York, NY: Routledge.

UNICEF. (2021). 5G-The misinformation which is still circulating. Retrieved from https://www.unicef.org/montenegro/en/stories/5g-technology-does-not-cause-or-spread-coronavirus

Verhoeven, P. (2016). The co-production of business news and its effects: The corporate framing mediated-moderation model. *Public Relations Review, 42*(4), 509–521. doi: 10.1016/j.pubrev.2016.03.006

Vos, T. P., & Russell, F. M. (2019). Theorizing journalism's institutional relationships: An elaboration of gatekeeping theory. *Journalism Studies, 20*(16), 2331–2348. doi:10.1080/1461670X.2019.1593882

Wang, C.-J., & Zhu, J. J. H. (2019). Jumping onto the bandwagon of collective gatekeepers: Testing the bandwagon effect of information diffusion on social news website. *Telematics and Informatics, 41*, 34–45.

4   Outbreak Communication

Introduction

Outbreak communication is communication that goes out to the public and different stakeholders as soon as a public health risk is known. The health-related messages at this stage focus on actions and behaviours that seek to prevent the spread of the disease and stop the outbreak. The fundamental purpose of outbreak communication is to provide timely information that is critical to alert other key stakeholders of a potential cross-border threat to public health. This is regarded as the most vital information which, when communicated early, will set national health authorities into higher levels of alertness and set into motion strategic choices that can enable containment of the disease at an early stage. Therefore, the health authorities at the outbreak source must alert the international community about an outbreak quickly. Communicating early and transparently can prevent a disease from escalating into an epidemic or pandemic. Outbreak communication is a proactive communication approach that allows the public health authorities and the public in general to adopt protective behaviours, increase disease surveillance, and allow for effective response preparation.

This chapter examines the challenges and dilemmas associated with outbreak communication. It argues that due to the potential seriousness of their consequences, outbreaks have to be communicated quickly to avert the spread of the disease and save lives. Timely sharing of information at the early stages of the outbreak can assist outbreak containment activities, whereas delays in communication can impede the response to the outbreak. While speed and early notification are crucial to the management of outbreaks, several factors hamper communication. These include the lack of complete scientific information upon which decisions should be based as well as the unpredictable nature of outbreaks, the fear of causing false alarms as well as political and economic interests. Transparency, early knowledge sharing, and communication of uncertainty are fundamental to managing the outbreak.

DOI: 10.4324/9781003401827-4

Timeliness of Outbreak Notifications

Timelines of notification is a critical element in outbreak management, as announcing the outbreak early prompts early response by public health authorities. Speed and timeliness of notification messages play a major role in the actions to prevent an outbreak from becoming an epidemic. Through proactive dissemination of information about infectious diseases, large-scale disease outbreaks can be prevented and stopped through early detection, notification, and rapid control. Time and again, public health authorities have underscored the vital importance of timely dissemination of risk-related information. Scientists have been using "timeliness" metrics to track the time from outbreak to detection and the time from detection to outbreak response. These metrics measure the time taken from the start of the outbreak to its detection, time to outbreak notification, and time to outbreak end. Figure 4.1 illustrates the time and stages to the outbreak end.

Notification is a result of a chain of events from infection to the time a report is registered with the local, national, and international public health services (Swaan, van den Broek, Kretzschmar, & Richardus, 2018). The speed between the steps is crucial for prompt intervention. Delays in the chain can have negative ramifications on the public health response. In their research on the timeliness of outbreak response in the WHO (World Health Organization) Africa Region between 2017 and 2019, Impouma et al. (2020) noted that there have been improvements in the systems to find, stop, and prevent epidemics. Out of the 296 outbreak cases in Africa, they noted that the time to detect disease and time to end the outbreak has decreased over the years, whereas the time to notify increased. It is this delay that is of concern. Delays in the notification can curtail international disease surveillance.

The COVID-19 pandemic is partially a consequence of delays in the chain and communication lapses in the timeliness of response. It indicates failure of measures to notify other public health services and to contain the outbreak in the geographical areas they occurred. In a highly mobile and interconnected world, characterized by intricate and faster networks of international travel, infectious diseases can reach different parts of the world in a relatively short time. Time is of the essence and so too are the early risk messages. The more the delay, the more the likelihood of the diseases spreading and even getting out of control.

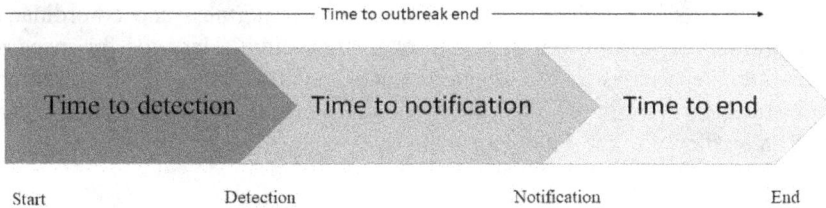

Figure 4.1 Timeliness in outbreak notification.

In their chronological analysis of how COVID-19 became a pandemic, an Independent Panel for Pandemic Preparedness and Response, while noting the dedicated response by WHO and some national governments, also show aspects of the response that *could have been quicker* and these include outbreak notifications (own emphasis) (Singh et al., 2021).

The WHO is responsible for the surveillance of threats to public health worldwide and its members have a responsibility to report to the body any "possible" threats they encounter in their territory. It has been noted that even though the coronavirus started spreading before December 2019, the Chinese authorities took a while before notifying WHO. Singh et al. (2021) note that outbreak response was curtailed at the beginning when the Wuhan Municipal Health Commission issued notices (with instructions not to share) to hospitals about cases of pneumonia of unknown origin in December 2020. The information was leaked to social media sites, where Li Wenliang and fellow doctors discussed the possibility of an outbreak. The initial response of the Wuhan authorities was to detain those "spreading rumours" of a possible outbreak and to dismiss the claims as false statements that disturbed the public order. According to Singh et al., reporting of the notices by the Chinese business publication *Finance Sina* triggered a chain of events that signalled the emergence of an outbreak, with WHO issuing a global alert on the outbreak on 5 January 2020. It further took another month of assessment before WHO declared the outbreak a Public Health Emergency of International Concern on 30 January. It took another few weeks before COVID-19 could be characterized as a pandemic.

There were significant delays in the chain of events. Time was lost while authorities in the disease management chain pondered on several questions to which no answers were readily known. Some of the delays are scientific, such as awaiting confirmation of laboratory results, while some are political, as noted above in the case of China. Not surprisingly, China has been blamed for being slow in their outbreak notification and for covering up the true scale of the crisis, as the source of the outbreak remains a mystery.[1] Some have blamed the WHO for not providing member countries with clear and timely information about the virus, while in other countries, the blame shifted to the national leaders ignoring messages from Beijing. Timelines in outbreak response mean timely and effective efforts in notifications to increase disease alertness and co-ordinated international response, given that the global risk is high. The need for speed in notifications continues to rise as international travel accelerates the movement of people. However, there are hurdles to be taken into consideration and some of these are explored in the following sections.

The 'Crying Wolf' Effect

Disease outbreaks have a higher degree of uncertainty and are very difficult to predict. No one knows for sure how an outbreak will unfold. Many outbreaks occur every year, but very few of these escalate into major health events.

Outbreaks are alarming for the public; they ignite fear and anxiety and create a huge demand for information. This is also the dilemma that confounds outbreak communications. Public authorities are doomed if they communicate early and cause needless panic or if they communicate late and lead to loss of life. Public authorities by nature are very cautious in giving out outbreak information lest they warn the public about a danger that does not eventuate. A dilemma that confounds public authorities during an outbreak is the fear of "crying wolf". In the fable *The Boy Who Cried Wolf*, a shepherd boy, who watched a flock of sheep near a village, brought the villagers out several times by shouting a false alarm "wolf, wolf". Realising that they have been duped, the villagers decided not to heed him any longer and therefore took no notice of his alarm when he actually needed their assistance. Because the villages did not see the wolf, they thought it did not exist; yet, it did.

In risk and emergency situations, recurring warnings about an event that then does not occur can lead to warning fatigue. The public gets desensitized to the threatened danger, thus endangering the risk communication efforts. A good example is weather warnings, where authorities have a dilemma when warning the public about the coming bad weather, based purely on scientific weather forecasts. Weather patterns can change leading to either reduced or enhanced threats. False alarms create a "cry wolf" effect, leading to the danger of the public ignoring the warnings.[2] Too many false alarms lead to inattention, complacency, and desensitization. Warning fatigue has been identified as one of the obstacles to effective emergency management in weather-related crises. To avoid creating false alarms, public authorities are sometimes hesitant to give warning messages, especially when there are doubts about the event happening.

Yet much of crisis and risk communication literature describe timeliness and effectiveness as being central to effective crisis management (Coombs, 2023; Reynolds & Seeger, 2005). A timely warning about an impending threat is seen as a precursor to the effectiveness of the crisis management effort. However, warning messages can mean different things, depending on the threat in question. Where full information is available and reliable, the warning can mean that the danger is real, it's happening, or arrival is certain. However, health warnings about severe disease outbreaks fall into the category of those crises where the danger is real, but there are uncertainties on how they would unfold. Disease notification is the most effective strategy for managing epidemic-prone outbreaks.

Transparency in Outbreak Communication

Transparency in communication is increasingly recognized as an important feature of risk and crisis management. Open and transparent public communication is a necessary prerequisite for the effective management of public health emergencies (O'Malley, Rainford, & Thompson, 2009). Lessons learned from previous epidemics and pandemics demonstrate that transparency and quick reactions can avert or minimize the rate and depth of spreading. Past pandemics such as the severe acute respiratory syndrome (SARS) and the 2009 influenza (H1N1) revealed several challenges and shortcomings in outbreak communications. The WHO described the SARS disease outbreak as a watershed event in terms of the impact that outbreaks might have in a closely connected world (WHO, 2005). The SARS travelled rapidly through routes of international travel, and within a short space of time, it had infected more than 8, 000 people worldwide. It showed world leaders the far-reaching consequences of an outbreak and the need to prioritize rapid public health response. It also highlighted the need to revisit outbreak communication. Outbreaks are no longer restricted to the local but have an international significance.

Drawing on experiences from the SARS outbreak of 2003, the WHO convened a summit in Kuala Lumpur, Malaysia, to ponder over the communication challenges often experienced during the past outbreaks (WHO, 2003). The summit recognized the need to sharpen outbreak communications to control the outbreaks faster, prevent them, and reduce their impact on society. It sought answers to two fundamental questions: first, on how communication could hasten containment; and second, on how communication could help mitigate the social and economic impact of the disease. The WHO summit identified five critical practices that influence the effectiveness of outbreak communication: building trust, announcing early, being transparent, respecting public concerns, and planning in advance (WHO, 2005).

Effective communication that integrates complete transparency forms the foundation of outbreak communication. The rationale for transparency has public health, strategic, and ethical dimensions (O'Malley et al., 2009). The WHO summit on SARS reaffirmed the need for transparency in outbreak messages: "Information should be communicated in a transparent, accurate and timely manner" (WHO, 2003). Timely and transparent communication with the public and the other stakeholders on the onset of an outbreak will engender co-operation in the efforts to prevent and stop the disease outbreak from escalating. Transparency is a key element in international co-ordination and collaboration. For a country or organization to be transparent, it means availability to the media, willingness to disclose information, and honesty (Coombs, 2019). Commitment to transparency should ideally underline the whole process of the outbreak response.

However, as O'Malley et al. (2009) note, there is a gap between rhetorical commitment and substantive action by public health authorities and governments. Transparency by public health authorities is not easy to track, conceptions of transparency vary, and assessments may be subjective. Drawing on interviews with WHO communication staff in public health emergencies between 2004 and 2008, O'Malley et al. (2009) noted that there were still persistent challenges that undermined transparency; these include: (a) reluctance to announce a potential threat until all information is scientifically confirmed and formally endorsed; (b) a tendency to withhold information that is potentially damaging to an economic sector; and (c) an emphasis on strict information control. The factors that undermine transparency in outbreak communications emanate from the involvement of political actors in crisis management and the economic considerations that weigh into the decision-making. As the experience of past and recent outbreaks has shown, "outbreak control and outbreak communication is rarely a pure, clean process of winning public trust and transmitting information objectively and openly. It is more often than not a messy business requiring political decisions with winners and losers" (Abraham, 2009a). More often, outbreak communication faces political leadership obstacles.

The Political Aspects of Outbreaks

Disease outbreaks have strong political dimensions. They are more than just public health events, and they occur "in a highly charged political, social and economic environment" (Abraham, 2011). The political context in which outbreaks occur shapes the nature of the outbreak communication challenges. Responses to the outbreaks are inherently political, bearing the influences of various actors at the local, national, regional, and global levels (McLean & Ewart, 2020). The political context shapes the narratives and the framing of the outbreak, given that they have far-reaching ramifications. Political authorities can impede outbreak control in their quest to protect other competing interests such as their political and economic interests. Given the wider implications of the outbreak, control measures, intrusion of the individual sphere, and economic losses can induce a loss of confidence in governments. Not surprisingly, an outbreak will undoubtedly grab the attention of the top echelons of government. WHO (2005) notes that such attention can be beneficial for outbreak communication "when it brings full political commitment to outbreak control, including adequate resources and high-level support for recommended interventions, even when these are costly and disruptive" (p. 8). WHO (2005) also noted that on the other end, "outbreak control can be severely impeded when officials decide to withhold information or downplay its significance". Opposition parties also are tempted to use the outbreak of an infectious disease for their benefit to gain political mileage. These are the political realities that challenge the ideal early announcement of outbreaks.

If political authorities are more motivated by economic interests rather than public health concerns, outbreak communication is likely to be impeded. A country's economic situation can be a leading factor in shaping outbreak communications. When long-term economic consequences are likely to follow the announcements of an outbreak, authorities at the outbreak source can be tempted to conceal or delay the information. For example, if there is an upcoming major event, authorities might downplay the outbreak to protect the economic, cultural, and political interests of that event. Japan faced a similar dilemma about the Tokyo 2020 Olympic Games. The country had invested heavily in infrastructure developments in preparation for the games. Besides the economic interests attached to hosting the games, the event was also of geo-strategic importance. Hence, despite the declaration of a global pandemic by the WHO, the Japanese government was persistent in holding the games in the summer of 2020. Even its Ministry of Health, Labour, and Welfare played a role in downplaying the pandemic. The event was eventually postponed. The conflict surrounding the postponement shows that health issues have strong political dimensions and political leadership can be tempted to play the economic card over the public safety card. The dilemma over competing choices impacts heavily outbreak communications as well.

During the avian influenza, since 2003, farmers in Asia faced a similar dilemma. Avian influenza is a highly contagious viral disease that affects chickens, turkeys, guinea fowls, and other birds. The outbreaks of avian influenza in the region continually threatened animal and public health, with extended consequences on the many livelihoods of the farmers and traders. Farmers depended on household chickens as an economic and food source; hence, voluntarily reporting sick birds would destroy their source of income unless they were compensated for the depopulated flocks (Takeuchi, 2006). Without compensation, the temptation to conceal the information by both the farmers and local leadership is greater than the risk of allowing the disease to spread. Abraham (2009a) refers to German sociologist Ulrich Beck's insights on the social and political basis of the notion of risk, and argues that the distribution of risk is never equitable but follows the unequal distribution of power in national societies as well as globally (ibid.). The way audiences perceive risk messages is dependent on their perception of risk distribution. Actors seeing themselves as bearing a disproportionate level of risk are likely not to comply and act for the benefit of public health. In global pandemics, there is often an uneven global distribution of the burden.

The issue of blame is central to the understanding of outbreaks and the attribution of responsibility to the causes and response to outbreaks. Several literature shows that there is a preponderance of cases where blame and responsibility are attributed to people's cultures (Kapiriri & Ross, 2020) or governments' actions. Authorities can be held accountable for the outbreak and hence might be tempted to conceal information about the outbreak for fear of being criticized. The attribution of responsibility to state actors and organizations also means responsibility to control the situation. It was reported in the media that the then US President Donald Trump wanted China to be held accountable for the losses and death caused by COVID-19. Speaking at a Republican Party convention in North Carolina, President Trump, referring COVID-19 as the "China virus", said that "China should pay USD10 trillion to America and the world, for the death and destruction they have caused".[3] Across the world, there was a growing chorus of voices calling for China to pay compensation for the damages caused by the virus. The fear of political blame and attribution of responsibility affect transparency in outbreak communications.

Unintended Consequences: Inform and Be Damned

Researchers in crisis communication emphasize the need to be quick with outbreak communication. A prompt notification can mitigate the spread of the disease. However, as experience shows, there are some unintended consequences for transparency and quick communications. The outbreak of the Omicron variant towards the end of 2021 provides a good example. When scientists in South Africa identified another variant of the coronavirus, they were quick to notify the world about this new mutation. The early announcement by South Africa of the outbreak of the SARS-CoV-2 Omicron variant while commendable from the perspective of the speed of outbreak communication, left South Africa bearing the economic consequences as foreign governments immediately introduced strict travel bans from the region. Even though the South African scientists who first detected the variant had claimed that their research so far indicated a much milder variant, the global response was to isolate the region. Those countries that imposed travel restrictions defended their proactive response on the need to prevent the spread of the new variant and to protect their citizens from the possible threat posed by Omicron. This proactive action was taken despite the lack of scientific data to support the decision. This is also another dilemma facing public health authorities, because waiting for scientific proof literally means allowing the disease to spread even further.

Political leaders in the affected regions of South Africa lamented the restrictions they viewed as being punitive and disproportionate to the threat. They argued that the restrictions would worsen their economies, which had already been battered by the pandemic. South African President Cyril Ramaphosa bemoaned the travel bans imposed on the region as being completely unjustified and discriminatory. Commenting on the Omicron backlash against Africa, WHO chief Tedros Adhanom Ghebreyesus noted that the reaction to South Africa's announcement of the outbreak was punitive rather than an expression of gratitude for detecting, sequencing, and promptly sharing the information about the new variant. He further argued that this reaction to an outbreak announcement "disincentivizes countries from alerting others to threats that will inevitably land on their shores" (ibid.). Health experts cautioned that the travel bans would set a harmful precedent. They would deter other countries from announcing outbreaks in their backyards for fear of backlash. A twitter comment by a handler identified as @ashishkjha captures this predicament in a tweet – "the signal to the next country is …if you identify a variant and share it with the global community you will be punished with a travel ban …" (6:28 p.m., 26 November 2021).

This echoes the view of South African epidemiologist Professor Salim Abdool Karim:

> The immediate reaction to the announcement of the variant was just outrageous and it was an overreaction … what it's basically saying to the rest of the world is that in future, if you have good surveillance systems and you have in

place the mechanisms to identify a new variant and to identify it early, then whatever you do, don't tell the world, keep it secret. Let some other country do the announcement so that you don't have to bear the burden of the reaction that we've had [to endure].

(Serino, 2021)

The statement captures the political predicament of outbreak communications. By announcing the outbreak of the new variant, South Africa took the economic burden on behalf of others. To use the analogy by Abraham (2009a) on the distribution of risk, South Africa is like a farmer with an outbreak of avian influenza on his farm and, from a public health perspective, needs to take on board a straightforward message to cull his chickens and ducks to curtail the outbreak. However, from the farmer's perspective, he is being asked to bear the costs of destroying his livelihood to reduce the risk to other members of society.

Co-ordination and Collaboration

Disease outbreaks need responsive and resilient systems of preparedness, management, and response. The risk of transmission elsewhere in the world and the perceived consequences for those affected attracts a lot of attention from different actors – all with different interests in the outbreak (Ndlela, 2019). In public health emergencies, risk of failure is shared across national boundaries, hence the need for collective action to mitigate the risk. The logic is a simple one – disease outbreaks know no boundaries. Outbreaks require extensive collaboration and co-ordination of public health authorities, governments, international governmental organizations, and non-governmental organizations at different levels – national, regional, and global levels. When multiple agencies respond to a disease outbreak, they need co-ordination – "the way organizations work together" (Bdeir, Hossain, & Crawford, 2013) – and collaboration – "the successful implementation of joint organized activities and procedures between private and public organizations" (Kim, Andrew, & Jung, 2017). In this context, maximization of communication messages between key stakeholders in various countries and across sectors is a prerequisite for success in outbreak response.

Communication messages are needed for efficient co-ordination and collaboration in public health response. It can be difficult to plan a response without adequate information. The quality of communication has a bearing on the effectiveness of co-ordination and collaboration. Effective communication involves openness and transparency in sharing or exchanging information between organizations and dissemination of information to the public about the nature of the outbreak. It also entails access to quality information. Changes in information-sharing mechanism, especially with the advent of digital communication and social media, mean that information on disease outbreaks can spread on social media even without the involvement of the organizations responsible, as shown in the case of the COVID-19 outbreak in China.

Managing risk information, regarding the outbreak and sharing that information with other stakeholders, is critical yet challenging in many ways. First, there are challenges associated with the very nature of the crisis risk, that is, the characteristics of disease outbreaks and the unpredictable nature of diseases, such as mutation possibilities and changes in the modes of transmission. Outbreaks are urgent public health conditions that require timely decisions to save lives and prevent further spread. However, decision-making is often compounded by the absence of solid scientific information during the outbreak. Without adequate scientific information to support decisions, outbreak communication can be delayed while experts scurry to make sense of the situation.

Outbreaks are very unpredictable and often occur in information-poor contexts. Likewise, when COVID-19 broke out in late 2019, very little information was known about the virus and its health risk, as it spread into different counties evolving into a pandemic despite various strategies to prevent the transmission. Second, information sharing is hampered by hierarchical organizational structures that impinge on horizontal co-ordination and information sharing across organizational boundaries. Governmental agencies often encounter issues of co-ordination in performing inter-jurisdictional activities (Kim et al., 2017). As Nelson et al. (2022) note, health sectors often remain siloed during non-outbreak periods, making collaboration and information sharing during outbreaks problematic.

Third, researchers have also pointed to the deterioration of the quality of information when many organizations are involved. This is based on the assumption that information gathering and dissemination is not a unilateral activity of one organization but multiple actors with different knowledge interests and biases. Discrepancies are likely to emerge between those organizations located in the centre of the networks and those in the peripheries. Inter-organizational collaboration during the coronavirus pandemic exposed the fractures in relationships. The current pandemic has highlighted the challenges of outbreak communication, co-ordination, and collaboration across sectors.

Perception of Risk

A common trait in the onset of outbreaks is that there are many competing voices in the outbreak phase. Just like a reporter's coverage of a story is immersed in cultural and political factors within his/her organization and the country, so too has been the understanding of the public health risk. Politicians have power in society and their speeches can affect risk perception by the public and influence support or even rejection of containment measures. The outbreak of the coronavirus was truncated by glaring contradictions as world leaders took different stances on the risk posed by the virus. An analysis of political speeches before and soon after the coronavirus was declared as a pandemic reveals ideological polarization in the manner in which world leaders responded to the outbreak.

In February 2020, the US president downplayed the warnings about the risk posed by the coronavirus. He equated it to a flu, something commonplace and not a threat to public health. "This is a flu. This is like a flu"[4] and "we've never closed down the country for the flu".[5] By comparing it to a flu, Trump minimized the threat and undoubtedly influenced the perception of many people globally. This comparison to a flu refuting science was repeated during the pandemic, culminating in Facebook and Twitter labelling the posts as misinformation and finally blocking them.

Following the announcement of the global pandemic by the WHO, Trump addressed the nation from the Oval Office on 11 March 2020. In the address, he informed the nation about the threat of a "foreign virus" and the need to take tough response measures to reduce the threat:

> This is the most aggressive and comprehensive effort to confront a foreign virus in modern history. I am confident that by counting and continuing to take these tough measures, we will significantly reduce the threat to our citizens, and we will ultimately and expeditiously defeat this virus.[6]

Trump emphasized that the threat was not new and that the US was ready to meet the challenging situation:

> From the beginning of time, nations and people have faced unforeseen challenges, including large-scale and very dangerous health threats. This is the way it always was and always will be. It only matters how you respond, and we are responding with great speed and professionalism.
>
> (ibid.)

The speech can also be analysed for the speaker's commitment to certain actions. This is a commissive speech act. According to Juniartha (2020), a commissive speech expresses the speaker's commitment to some future action. Promises, guarantees, refusal, and threats are key elements of commissive speech acts. Trump promises new measures to prevent the infections from spreading. He underlies the commitment the US government will take to stem the infections. The measures include restricting and suspending travel from China, Europe, and other hotspots. He undertakes "strong but necessary actions to protect the health and wellbeing of all Americans". In the speech, he discredits the EU for failing to take the same precautions and as a result, a large number of new clusters in the US were seeded by travellers from Europe. There is an apportionment of blame in the speech.

However, despite the commitment to action, Trump expressively downplays the risk posed by the coronavirus, claiming that to most Americans *"the risk is very, very low"* (own emphasis). This conclusion is not supported by any research and appears to undermine drastic measures being put in place. As noted by Kakisina et al. (2022), Trump "appears to underestimate the severity of the threat faced by the country, contradicting his previous action of calling a national emergency on the virus" (p. 4). The actions of the Trump administration sent mixed measures about the real extent of the risk, including undermining science and undermining recommendations from the Centers for Disease Control and Prevention (CDC). Trump "knowingly downplayed the coronavirus, even though he knew it was more deadly than a seasonal flu",[7] something he acknowledges in a conversation with *The Washington Post* journalist Bob Woodward.[8]

Another political leader who has downplayed the coronavirus is Brazilian President Jair Bolsonaro. On 24 March 2020, in an address to the nation, Bolsonaro compared the coronavirus to a "little flu", and barely two months after that comment more than 132,000 cases of COVID-19 were registered in Brazil.[9] This was followed by similar statements and actions trivialising the coronavirus despite the increasing infections and deaths in Brazil. Dismissing the risk posed by the coronavirus, the Brazilian president proceeded to defy WHO recommendations for social distancing, lockdown, and isolation and urged his country to remain open. Similarly, in Tanzania, muddled messages about the outbreak hampered the country's preparedness and response. The then-Tanzanian President John Magufuli repeatedly minimized the risk of COVID-19, resulting in confusing messages. "He ignored scientific reason – championing religious devotion" in his response to the pandemic.[10]

Mixed messages and downplaying of the coronavirus outbreak affected critical aspects of the global response, resulting in chaos and confusion. In a context with multiple information intermediaries, there are dangers of different perceptions of the outbreak and hence contradictory messages about it. As noted above, public authorities can downplay the seriousness of the outbreak to protect other interests, be it political or economic interests.

Conclusion

This chapter has highlighted the importance of outbreak communication. Outbreak communication is crucial for rapid responses to the outbreak of infectious diseases. Timely and transparent communication from the outbreak source is essential to aiding decision-making, co-ordination, and collaboration among various levels of public agencies and other actors during a public health crisis. Successful communication with the public during an outbreak can encourage the public to adopt behaviours that can contribute to threat reduction.

However, outbreak communication is often clouded with uncertainty from the onset. Without full scientific proof, the full threat of the outbreak is not known. The consequence is that vital information may be silenced or might drown while authorities wait for verification of information. Abraham (2009b) notes that if messages are drowned out, distorted, or ignored by competing social voices, then outbreak communication will not achieve its public health goal of helping prevent and control outbreaks. He argues that in such a situation, communication strategists need to strive towards two goals. First, they must strive for visibility, that is, the ability to get the message across clearly and prominently to the public and not be drowned by competing voices. Visibility can be achieved by choosing the best channel of communication and the right spokesperson. Second, legitimacy – ensuring that information is seen as legitimate and authoritative. The coronavirus pandemic has highlighted the challenges of uncoordinated outbreak messages and approaches to responding to the outbreak.

The COVID-19 pandemic brought to the fore fragmentation of the public emergence ecosystem, that is, "the institutions, leadership and governance structures, mechanisms, frameworks, policies, actors and stakeholders that contribute to global health emergency preparedness and response" (GPMB, 2021). Muddled outbreak communication messages led to polarization, challenged science, and generally thwarted a unified global response to the threat as envisaged in the WHO conference in Kuala Lumpur. Risk and communication messages during the COVID-19 outbreak complicated the responses around the world.

Notes

1 https://www.express.co.uk/news/world/1271028/Angela-Merkel-Germany-China-coronavirus-blame-Wuhan-Xi-Jinping-Trump-latest (Accessed 19.04.2020).
2 https://www.bushfirecrc.com/news/news-item/crying-wolf-myths-warning-fatigue (see notes).
3 https://www.ndtv.com/india-news/china-dismisses-donald-trumps-10-trillion-compensation-for-covid-spread-2458517 (Accessed 05.05.2022).
4 https://www.forbes.com/sites/tommybeer/2020/09/10/all-the-times-trump-compared-covid-19-to-the-flu-even-after-he-knew-covid-19-was-far-more-deadly/?sh=46a3487cf9d2 (Accessed 09.05.2022).
5 https://www.france24.com/en/20200401-now-trump-says-it-s-wrong-to-compare-coronavirus-to-regular-flu (Accessed 09.05.2022).
6 https://trumpwhitehouse.archives.gov/briefings-statements/remarks-president-trump-address-nation/ (Accessed 09.05.2022).
7 https://www.npr.org/sections/latest-updates-trump-covid-19-results/2020/10/02/919432383/how-trump-has-downplayed-the-coronavirus-pandemic (Accessed 09.05.2022).
8 https://www.forbes.com/sites/tommybeer/2020/09/10/all-the-times-trump-compared-covid-19-to-the-flu-even-after-he-knew-covid-19-was-far-more-deadly/?sh=46a3487cf9d2 (Accessed 09.05.2022).
9 https://edition.cnn.com/2020/05/08/americas/brazil-coronavirus-bolsonaro-response-intl/index.html (Accessed 09.05.2022).
10 https://www.csis.org/analysis/implications-tanzanias-bungled-response-covid-19 (Accessed 09.05.2022).

References

Abraham, T. (2009a). Risk and outbreak communication: Lessons from alternative paradigms. *Bulletin of the World Health Organization, 87*(8), 604–607. doi:10.2471/blt.08.058149

Abraham, T. (2009b). Risk and outbreak communication: Lessons from alternative paradigms. *Bulletin,* 604–607. https://www.scielosp.org/pdf/bwho/2009.v87n8/604-607. doi:10.2471/BLT.08.058149

Abraham, T. (2011). Lessons from the pandemic: The need for new tools for risk and outbreak communication. *Emerging Health Threats Journal, 4*(1), 7160. doi:10.3402/ehtj.v4i0.7160

Bdeir, F., Hossain, L., & Crawford, J. (2013). Emerging coordination and knowledge transfer process during disease outbreak. *Knowledge Management Research & Practice, 11*(3), 241–254. doi:10.1057/kmrp.2012.1

Coombs, W. T. (2019). *Ongoing Crisis Communication: Planning, Managing, and Responding* (5 ed.). Los Angeles, CA: Sage.

Coombs, W. T. (2023). *Ongoing Crisis Communication. Planning, Managing, and Responding* (6 ed.). Thousand Oaks, CA: Sage.

GPMB. (2021). From worlds apart to a world prepared. Retrieved from https://www.gpmb.org/docs/librariesprovider17/default-document-library/gpmb-annual-report-2021.pdf?sfvrsn=44d10dfa_9

Impouma, B., Roelens, M., Williams, G., Flahault, A., Codeço, C., Moussana, F., & Keiser, O. (2020). Measuring timeliness of outbreak response in the World Health Organization African region, 2017–2019. *Emerging Infectious Diseases, 26*(11), 2555–2564. doi:10.3201/eid2611.191766

Juniartha, I. W. (2020). Commissive Speech act in the movie John Wick Chapter 2. *Lingual: Journal of Language and Culture, 10*(2). doi:10.24843/LJLC.2020.v10.i02.p06

Kakisina, P. A., Indhiarti, T. R., & Al Fajri, M. S. (2022). Discursive strategies of manipulation in COVID-19 political discourse: The case of Donald Trump and Jair Bolsonaro. *SAGE Open, 12*(1), 21582440221079884. doi:10.1177/21582440221079884

Kapiriri, L., & Ross, A. (2020). The politics of disease epidemics: A Comparative analysis of the SARS, Zika, and Ebola outbreaks. *Global Social Welfare, 7*(1), 33–45. doi:10.1007/s40609-018-0123-y

Kim, K., Andrew, S. A., & Jung, K. (2017). Public health network structure and collaboration effectiveness during the 2015 MERS outbreak in South Korea: An Institutional Collective Action Framework, *14*(9), 1064.

McLean, H., & Ewart, J. (2020). *Political Leadership in Disaster and Crisis Communication and Management: International Perspectives and Practices*. Cham, Switzerland: Palgrave Macmillan.

Ndlela, M. (2019). *Crisis Communication: A Stakeholder Perspective*. Cham, Switzerland: Palgrave Macmillan.

Nelson, S., Abimbola, S., Jenkins, A., Naivalu, K., & Negin, J. (2022). Information sharing, collaboration, and decision-making during disease outbreaks: The experience of Fiji. *Journal of Decision Systems, 31*(1–2), 171–188. doi:10.1080/12460125.2021.1927486

O'Malley, P., Rainford, J., & Thompson, A. (2009). Transparency during public health emergencies: From rhetoric to reality. *Bulletin of the World Health Organization, 87*(8), 614–618. doi:10.2471/blt.08.056689

Reynolds, B., & Seeger, M. W. (2005). Crisis and emergency risk communication as an integrative model. *Journal of Health Communication, 10*(1), 43–55.

Serino, K. (2021). Travel bans punish countries for doing necessary work to end the pandemic, South Africa epidemiologist says. https://www.pbs.org/newshour/health/outrageous-and-an-overreaction-south-africas-top-epidemiologist-responds-to-omicron-travel-ban

Singh, S., McNab, C., Olson, R. M., Bristol, N., Nolan, C., Bergstrøm, E., . . . Phelan, A. (2021). How an outbreak became a pandemic: A chronological analysis of crucial junctures and international obligations in the early months of the COVID-19 pandemic. *The Lancet, 398*(10316), 2109–2124. doi:10.1016/S0140-6736(21)01897-3

Swaan, C., van den Broek, A., Kretzschmar, M., & Richardus, J. H. (2018). Timeliness of notification systems for infectious diseases: A systematic literature review. *PLOS ONE, 13*(6), e0198845–e0198845. doi:10.1371/journal.pone.0198845

Takeuchi, M. T. (2006). Avian influenza risk communication, Thailand. *Emerging Infectious Diseases, 12*(7), 1172–1173. doi:10.3201/eid1207.060277

WHO. (2003). *Global Conference on Severe Acute Respiratory Syndrome (SARS): Where Do We Go from Here? (Summary Report)*. 17-18 June 2003, Kuala Lumpur (Malaysia). Available at Weekly Epidemiological Record *78*(34), 299–303.

WHO. (2005). *Outbreak Communication: Best Practices for Communicating with the Public during an Outbreak* (WHO/CDS/2005.32). Retrieved from https://www.who.int/publications/i/item/outbreak-communication-best-practices-for-communicating-with-the-public-during-an-outbreak (Accessed 21.06.2023).

5   Lockdown Messages

Introduction

As the number of infected people increased exponentially, the coronavirus erupted into a full-scale pandemic. Mathematical models predicted huge numbers of infections and hospitalization. There were concerns that the pandemic would affect the national health system's capacity to effectively handle patients, especially those that require intensive treatment at the same time. The exponential growth curves indicated that the pandemic would soon overweigh national health capacities. The epidemic curves, that is, the statistical charts visualizing the new infection cases, all pointed towards a dire peak situation, where the numbers of people gasping for oxygen in the intensive care units would surpass the available resources such as respirator equipment and protective gear. It would only be a matter of time before national health capacities were overwhelmed. In the absence of medication against the coronavirus, three different measures to counteract the emergency emerged, namely (i) vaccination, (ii) herd immunity development, and (iii) lockdown (Migliaccio, Buono, Maltese, & Migliaccio, 2021). Given that the first measure was not ready in the early stages of the pandemic and that vaccine development is a slow process, countries had to weigh in on options two and three. While few countries like Sweden opted for herd immunity development, regarded by some as being irresponsible, an overwhelming majority of countries opted for the third option of lockdown, despite its controversy and adverse economic effects.

The COVID-19 pandemic sent shockwaves throughout the world, as panic-stricken public health authorities set into action lockdown policy measures trying to mitigate the effect of the spread. One country after another went into various forms of unprecedented "lockdowns", ostensibly to "flatten the curve". The overarching goal of the lockdown measures was to control and contain COVID-19 by slowing down and reducing the infection rate and thereby flattening the epidemic curve. Lockdowns denote various forms of preventive measures and requirements that restrict the movement of people during an emergency such as public health concern, terrorist attack, or riot. Even though the concept

DOI: 10.4324/9781003401827-5

was widely used during the pandemic, there is no clear-cut definition. Haider et al. (2020) define lockdown as "a set of measures aimed at reducing transmission of COVID-19 that are mandatory, applied indiscriminately to a general population and involve some restrictions on the established pattern of social and economic life" (p. 2). As an emergency protocol, lockdowns prevent people from entering or leaving designated areas due to specific risks that can harm them or others if they move freely (such as COVID-19). The primary objective of a lockdown during a public health concern is to restrict the transmission from person to person, to isolate those infected or likely to be infected, and to physical distance to avoid exposure to an infectious disease. In the absence of medical interventions, lockdown measures help contain or delay the spread of communicable diseases like COVID-19. The main goal of the intervention is to break the chain of infection and delay the rate of new infections. Delaying the transmissions allow society to prepare adequately and to maintain the structure and capacity of the existing infrastructure.

Lockdowns can be full, partial, or limited. *Full lockdown* usually means that populations in the specified area must stay where they are and may not leave the area (geographical containment). In extreme cases, people are not even allowed to leave their homes (stay-at-home), except when going to buy food and medicines. *Partial lockdown* is less severe than full lockdown, in that it can allow services to be open within specific periods, for example, bars, restaurants, and cafes can close early evenings. The concepts "hard" or "soft" have also been used to denote the type of lockdown. *Preventive lockdown* is taken as a preventive measure to mitigate risk, for example, by limiting travellers from red zone countries and regions.

While lockdowns are effective and valuable measures during disease outbreaks, their implementation is subject to resistance. Hence, lockdowns must be supplemented by extensive public health communications, more particularly instructional information, telling the public what to do and explaining why they should do as requested. Lockdown measures are sometimes, if not often, considered controversial and very intrusive on individual rights. Many researchers have noted that quarantine measures raise several legal, social, financial, and logistical challenges (Rothstein et al., 2003; Tognotti, 2013). These strategic measures have several political, economic, social, and ethical implications, and hence are prone to intense debates and polarization. The measures are sometimes met with scepticism, suspicion, and even outright rejection by sections of the public who consider them an infringement of their rights. As such, as Rothstein et al. (2003) argue, "obtaining and maintaining public trust are key to the successful implementation of these measures". Clear messages about the criteria and justification for and the role and duration of quarantine will help generate public trust. At the same time, it should be noted that public trust is not something that can be established overnight. Where there is little trust, compliance would be compromised. Correct messages alone are not enough in the absence of trust.

The main objective of this chapter is to examine, through case studies, lockdown messages communicated during the early periods of national lockdowns. It analyses the strategies employed and the language used in informing the public of the drastic measures. This chapter also ponders on the effectiveness and lack of effectiveness in these initial communications. It explores the challenges faced by governments in lockdown communications and how these were overcome. All communication that happens in the outbreak stages of a pandemic set the premise for further communication management during the crisis.

Lockdown: Revisiting Centuries-Old Strategies

In most countries around the world, the initial response to the COVID-19 risk was through a variety of lockdown strategies. Since March 2019, various forms of lockdowns were implemented across the world, and by the end of April 2020, an estimated half of the world population was under some form of lockdown. Lockdowns and quarantines have for centuries become a vital public health tool for combating epidemics and pandemics. Physical distancing, isolation, and movement restrictions are not a new phenomenon. The measures can be traced back to ancient societies before the prevalence of pharmaceutical interventions like drugs and vaccines. In biblical times, sufferers of leprosy were isolated for a certain period to avoid contact with other people. In traditional African communities, the sick were banished from the community for a certain period. In medieval Europe, sufferers of leprosy were forced to wear distinctive clothes and compelled to announce their presence with bells. This was intended to warn others to keep their distance and avoid any close contact that could increase the possibility of transmission. The fourteenth-century bubonic plague pandemic in Europe, also known as the Black Death, witnessed pandemic response measures that are akin to *quarantine*. In a broader sense, the quarantine strategy involves measures to separate persons, animals, and goods that may have been exposed to a contagious disease (Tognotti, 2013).

In an article entitled *Lessons from the History of Quarantine, from Plague to Influenza A*, Tognotti (2013) provides a historical perspective of the strategy of quarantine, starting as far back as the plague epidemic of 1347–1352 to the twenty-first-century outbreaks such as the SARS pandemic (2003) and the 2009 Influenza A (HINI). The responses to the plagues are regarded as the first organized institutional responses to disease control. As medicine was impotent against the plague, the only way then to escape infection was to avoid contact with infected persons and contaminated objects (Tognotti, 2013). For example, city-states or nations prevented strangers from entering their territories. They did so by deploying armed guards or military on access points to the cities or on transit routes.

During the COVID-19 pandemic, the centuries-old strategy of lockdown was revisited in the public health response. The term lockdown was used for a variety of mass quarantines, shutdowns, shelter-in-place, and stay-at-home orders. Preventive lockdowns are pre-emptive measures to mitigate the risk of person-to-person infections. By limiting the movement of people, authorities aimed at slowing down the rate of infection and rebalancing health resources. Hence people were ordered to stay at home, work from home, keep social distancing, and avoid unnecessary travel. National borders were partially or fully closed to prevent people from coming in or leaving. Airlines were grounded as passenger numbers dwindled due to the closure of national borders. Except for specified essential services such as food retail, transportation, manufacturing, security, and health sectors, the lockdown saw several non-essential services shutting down. Schools, colleges, and universities hurriedly moved to online teaching, while restaurants and bars closed their doors.

The second strategy involved quarantine, that is, "the separation and restriction of movement or activities of persons who are not ill but who are believed to have been exposed to infection, for the purpose of preventing transmission of diseases" (Rothstein et al., 2003). People can be quarantined in their homes or any designated facilities. Travellers arriving from areas with higher infection rates were quarantined. Large-scale quarantines were used in many countries during the 2003 SARS outbreak. In the context of the containment of COVID-19, the World Health Organization (WHO) issued guidelines for the quarantine of individuals (WHO, 2021).

The third strategy is isolation, that is, "the separation and restriction of movement or activities of infected persons who have a contagious disease, for the purpose of preventing transmission to others" (Rothstein et al., 2003). This strategy involved a rigid separation of healthy and infected persons. For example, passengers and crew disembarking ships were detained in makeshift camps for a period. Hospitals or care centres for the sick were placed far enough away from the populated areas. This strategy has become a powerful component of public health response to emerging and re-emerging infectious diseases.

Lockdown Messages. Adherence, Compliance, and Non-Compliance

Lockdown messages, as the name denotes, are a form of communication campaign intended for specific outcomes in a given area, within a specified period, in connection with a lockdown restriction. In public health, crisis authorities might try to limit movement in specified areas due to outbreaks of infections in those areas. The objective of these measures is to slow down or limit the spread of the disease from one area to another. The objective can also mean isolating areas where infections have been reported. During the pandemic, we witnessed different forms of lockdowns, be it full or partial lockdowns, and these had to be communicated to the intended audiences, locally, regionally, and internationally. The type of lockdown informs the selection of communication types, messages, and channel usage.

Haider et al. (2020) divide the lockdown messages into two main categories. The first category of measures includes message types that seek voluntary compliance by the targeted or general population. The messages are advisory in nature and offer a set of recommendations and behaviours, including hygiene measures, physical distancing, isolation or quarantine, and avoidance of gatherings and crowded places (ibid.). The second category of measures includes messages that require compulsory actions and behaviours. The messages target similar behavioural requirements. The difference is that non-compliance is punishable by law. For example, if gatherings are prohibited, non-compliance might incur a penalty fine or imprisonment.

The intended audiences in a lockdown are those earmarked for the lockdown action plan. It can be target individuals (or identifiable groups) or the general population. The intended audiences for lockdown messages are populations within specified geographical areas, be it a city, region, or the entire country that the authorities seek to place on lockdown. Message efficiency is achieved if the public authorities manage to get the messages across to the intended audiences, and the message produces intended responses, adherence, and compliance with the recommendations.

Adherence to the message means that the intended audience adopts appropriate behavioural changes that are in lieu with the intended outcomes. Adherence is an active choice compared to compliance, where the intended audience simply does as they are being told. Achieving adherence and compliance to lockdown measures require conceited communication focus and persuasive appeals. Effective communication and audience predisposition can eliminate or minimize the risk of deviation – intentional or unintentional. The choice of message types to support the lockdown actions is hence crucial to the success of the measures. Good communication can motivate the public to adopt risk-averting behaviours, for example, by staying in their homes.

Message Types

Four types of messages can be used in lockdown communications:

- *Educational messages*: These are messages that seek to educate the public about the disease so that they have enough knowledge to make educated decisions about how best to protect themselves and their families against the disease. These messages seek to provide scientific facts about the disease: what it is and how it spread.
- *Awareness messages*: These are messages that seek to raise public awareness about the disease (i.e. coronavirus) and also inform the target populations about the scope, nature, and duration of lockdown measures in their area. Ideally, these messages should be customized and targeted to the intended audiences.

- *Instructional messages*: These are messages that seek to tell intended populations what to do to protect themselves from the coronavirus. During a lockdown, the primary objective of the messages is to instruct the public to remain within certain boundaries. For example, messages can direct people to shelter-in-place, that is, seek safety within the building/home that one already occupies because of the imminent risk outside. The public is directed to stay indoors unless it is necessary to leave (e.g. to seek food and medication). Messages can also inform people to self-isolate.
- *Persuasive messages*: These are messages that purposely seek to influence people to adopt certain behaviours, such as staying at home, avoiding unnecessary travel, and comply with lockdown policy measures. Unlike instructional messages, persuasive messages can occur at a very low level of awareness or even unconsciously.

Communicators should anticipate several reactions to these messages, with audiences responding as intended with adherence and compliance or with people not complying with the messages. Audience predisposition, for example, what the audience already knows about the topic, their values, and attitudes, and current health behaviours play an important role in determining the responses (Salmon & Atkin, 2003). The environment and cultural context are some of the factors that influence the overall outcomes of the lockdown messages.

The COVID-19 lockdown created an unprecedented demand for public health communication messages. The impending lockdowns tested the communication abilities of leaders globally, as one after the other informed their bewildered, fearful, and sceptical audience that the nation was going to lockdown modus. This challenged leaders to demonstrate communication skills, be it persuasion, dialogue, or direct orders. They had to unequivocally convince people that their freedom of movement had been withdrawn and they should stay at home. Government officials and public health experts struggled with the aspect of finding a proper balance in the tone and style of their communication messages. The choice of language used by the leaders was critical in whether the people would adhere to and comply with the messages or not. Many variables affect the public response to strategic measures like lockdowns, isolation, and quarantine. The degree of trust in public authorities, national and sub-national cultures, and social factors bear in the reception of lockdown measures and also in the choice of lockdown variants. Voluntary adherence to lockdown measures presupposes that the public hears the messages and responds as expected. According to Rothstein et al. (2003), "isolation and quarantine are optimally performed on a voluntary basis, in accordance with instructions of healthcare providers and health officials".

The following case studies examine how leaders in selected countries communicated with their citizens and how audiences responded to the lockdown messages.

Case Studies

Many countries chose a variety of lockdown measures to contain the spread of COVID-19. Countries have differed in their approaches to the enforcement of lockdown measures, ranging from partial to full lockdown. By April 2020, a third of the world population was in some form of coronavirus lockdown, with their movement controlled and restricted by respective governments (Buchholz, 2020). One of the biggest lockdowns was enforced in India, where the government ordered 1.3 billion people to stay inside for 21 days, thus exceeding the number of Chinese placed on lockdown even at the height of the epidemic there. Most states in the US enforced strict stay-at-home orders, while in Europe more than 300 million people faced restricted movements. In Latin America, over 200 million people were locked down. The strategies for lockdown varied immensely from country to country. In some countries, the lockdowns were enforced through various forms of persuasion and laws (including draconian laws), while others derived from police and military enforcement. This section provides a case study of lockdowns in selected countries.

South Africa's *Thuma Mina*

Four speeches on the first nationwide lockdown are presented and analysed in this case study. These are speeches made by President Ramaphosa on 15, 23, and 26 March 2020. The messages in these speeches indicate shifting strategies from persuasive appeals to cohesive measures backed by security forces. The war discourse permeates most of the speeches, evoking national unity, resistance, war, defence, and victory over the virus.

Appeal – "The Most Definitive Thuma Mina *Moment"*

On 15 March 2020, President Cyril Ramaphosa (2020)[1] addressed the nation on the coronavirus pandemic, using both rational and emotional appeals in the speech. He briefed the nation about the impending crisis and what it meant for South Africa:

> The world is facing a medical emergency far graver than what we have experienced in over a century. The World Health Organisation has declared the coronavirus outbreak as a global pandemic... Given the scale and the speed at which the virus is spreading, it is now clear that no country is immune from the disease or will be spared its severe impact. Never before in the history of our democracy has our country been confronted with such a severe situation.
>
> (Ramaphosa, 2020)

Given the gravity of the situation as evidenced by the growing number of people (more than 162,000) that have tested positive for the coronavirus across the globe, this "calls for an extraordinary response". He underscores the justifications for the measures by providing references to statistical information that appeal to reasoning or logic (*logos*). Ramaphosa went on to outline a series of measures that the South African government was putting into place to protect the citizens and mitigate the risk:

> We have decided to take urgent and drastic measures to manage the disease, protect the people of our country and reduce the impact of the virus on our society and on our economy. We have now declared a national state of disaster in terms of the Disaster Management Act.

Invoking the state of disaster legislation would enable the government to mobilize resources, integrate and co-ordinate disaster management mechanisms. This will also enable the government to set up emergency, rapid, and effective response systems to mitigate the severity of its impact. The president also outlined the rolling out of a mass communication campaign on good hygiene and effective prevention behaviour. He made it clear that the contagious virus would be extremely disruptive to the "day-to-day life of our society". The president made an emotional appeal to all South Africans to stand together in solidarity and work together for a common cause. Everyone can participate and contribute to halting the transmission through a "change of behaviour amongst all South Africans" and "collectively" they can limit the effects of the disease:

> We are responding as a united nation to a common threat. This national emergency demands cooperation, collaboration and common action. More than that, it requires solidarity, understanding and compassion. Those who have resources, those who are healthy, need to assist those who are in need and who are vulnerable.

The president also tries to allay the fear – "we must accept the anxiety that it causes, but we cannot allow ourselves to be overwhelmed by fear and panic".

In concluding his statement, the President evoked a popular traditional church lyric, *thuma mina* (translates to send me). He defines the crisis as "the most definitive *Thuma Mina* moment for our country" and is hopeful that the people would respond positively to this call to common action. The phrase *thuma mina* is drawn from the Bible: "Then I heard the voice of the Lord saying, 'Whom shall I send? And who will go for us?' And I said, 'Here am I. Send me!'" (Isaiah, 6:8). The phrase, commonly used in church songs, was also popularized in a song by the famous South African musician, the late Hugh Masekela. The phrase was extensively used during the struggles against the apartheid regime.

As such, *thuma mina* has deeper political and cultural meanings in the South African context. As Maluleke (2018) notes, it calls for "self-sacrifice, individual responsibility and the importance of personal change in mindset" (Maluleke, 2018). It can be argued that the president's speech resonated well with the majority black audience, and was very inspirational and emotionally arousing. Atkin (2001) notes that to influence behaviour, the presentation should be personally involving and relevant, such that the receivers regard the recommendation as applicable to their situation and needs. By drawing on well-known culturally relevant lyrics, the president connected with the receivers. In his address to the parliament, President Ramaphosa acknowledged that many South Africans sent him messages consisting of only two words, *thuma mina* (send me).

Shift to a Discourse of War

The *thuma mina* moment was short-lived as the South African government moved away from the persuasive appeal messages to the discourse of war. The war discourse refers to the use of war language and rhetoric in the representation of the coronavirus pandemic. It uses language to personalize the virus as an enemy to be fought and defeated and legitimize actions associated with war. These actions and measures are made to appear appropriate, justifiable, and reasonable, given the warlike situation. The rhetoric of war permeates much of the president's speech and actions leading to the declaration of a nationwide lockdown. As Mawere (2020) notes, "as concerns about COVID-19's 'threat' to the nation grew, there is a clear trajectory where Ramaphosa's language and approaches move from medical interventions and management, national welfarism, and economic cushioning, to military and combatant language and approaches". The language of war is used to psychologically prepare the public for the great war against the virus.

On 23 March 2020, barely a week after the first *thuma mina* speech, the president set the setting for a militarized response:

> It is a week since we declared the coronavirus pandemic a national disaster and announced a package of extraordinary measures to combat this grave public health emergency. The response of the South African people to this crisis has been remarkable. Millions of our people have understood the gravity of the situation. Most South Africans have accepted the restrictions that have been placed on their lives and have taken responsibility for changing their behaviour … Many have had to make difficult choices and sacrifices, but all have been determined that these choices and sacrifices are absolutely necessary if our country is to emerge stronger from this disaster.

President Ramaphosa refers to the experience of other countries and how they have responded to the crisis and succeeded in slowing the transmission. With this, he set the tone to justify the impending lockdown to be enforced by the police and the military forces:

> We have learnt a great deal from the experiences of other countries. Those countries that have acted swiftly and dramatically have been far more effective in controlling the spread of the disease.

The president provides a justification to enforce a nationwide lockdown for 21 days with effect from midnight on Thursday 26 March 2020. The President calls for individual sacrifices. To save lives, it is necessary to disrupt everyday life:

> This is a decisive measure to save millions of South Africans from infection and save the lives of hundreds of thousands of people. While this measure will have a considerable impact on people's livelihoods, on the life of our society and on our economy, the human cost of delaying this action would be far, far greater.

The president then sets the tone for the militarized approach:

> The nation-wide lockdown is necessary to fundamentally disrupt the chain of transmission across society. I have accordingly directed the South African National Defence Force be deployed to support the South African Police Service in ensuring that the measures we are announcing are implemented.

Aware that the general public would not adhere to or comply with the lockdown messages, the government changed the strategy, leaning more towards a compulsory and mandatory approach through a militarized law-and-order framework (Seekings & Nattrass, 2020). The minister of the police was given unprecedented powers (ibid.) The rhetoric shifted towards the militarization of the COVID-19 response.

Militarized Lockdown

On 26 March 2020, a few days after the national lockdown was announced, President Ramaphosa appeared in full military regalia, when he addressed the South African National Defence Force (SANDF) ahead of their deployment to go out and wage the war against an invisible enemy – COVID-19 under a mission dubbed "Mission Save Lives":

> I am dressed in your uniform as your commander-in-chief to signify my support and solidarity with you as you embark on this most important mission in the history of our country.

There is symbolism in the president's attire, representing his role as head of the military, which was being deployed to fight the enemy. The country is facing an enemy that must be fought and defeated. "We will wage war against the invisible enemy, coronavirus. You are expected, as soldiers of the RSA, to defend our people against this virus. Your mission is to save lives". "A soldier swears they are going to do everything to do what's right for the people of South Africa", he said. "We must implement this very tough decision to lockdown South Africa and allow only minimal movement. The infection rate has now reached 927 and in a few days, we could be at 1,500. Our task is to minimise this infection rate".

The government initially deployed 2,820 soldiers, but this number increased to more than 70,000 within three weeks, making the biggest-ever deployment of the SANDF (Bester, Els, & Olivier, 2020). The lockdown enforced by the security forces can be viewed as a proactive action to minimize the risk of the coronavirus to public health, in a context where communication campaigns alone were seen as ineffective. The war imagery dominated the South African lockdown measures. Despite the president's plea to soldiers to act with kindness and compassion, the enforcement quickly turned brutal resulting in the loss of life and injuries. Images of soldiers patrolling the streets and imposing martial punishment to enforce the lockdown circulated the social media platforms. The campaign used fear to compel the citizens to comply with the strict lockdown measures. The punitive enforcement of the lockdown measures through a militarized response exacerbated the conditions of the less privileged, in a country marked with an extremely uneven distribution of wealth, power and privilege. Even with these staggering numbers, the security forces struggled to enforce them.

Why Lockdown Couldn't Work

The key lockdown message in Ramaphosa's speeches was that South Africans in all sectors, except those in the critical sectors, were to stay at home. Individuals would not be allowed to leave their homes during the lockdown, except when going to buy essentials like grocery shopping and medical care. Seekings and Nattrass (2020) note that the restrictions announced by President Ramaphosa were strict and early, commencing the same day the country recorded its first death from COVID-19. The lockdown level 5 announced by the government was one of the world's strictest, with the closure of all non-essential business and a ban on alcohol or cigarettes, jogging or dog-walking.

In the article *Lockdown didn't work in South Africa: Why it shouldn't happen again*, Smart et al. (2020) show that data concerning both the spread of the virus and the indirect consequences of the lockdown suggest that the severe restrictions imposed in South Africa were far from effective. They argue that it was easy to see from the beginning that the lockdown would be unfeasible in much of South Africa. They note that "overcrowded conditions, reliance on social grants and food parcels for which queuing is necessary, and shared ablutions all substantially change the effect of a regulation that says, 'stay at home'" (Smart, Broadbent, and Combrink, 2020). The effectiveness of the message is curtailed by the context that makes social distancing difficult. The contextual conditions of the people living in South Africa and in Africa in general mean that lockdown strategies were unlikely to be effective because they were devoid of context.

South Africa is one of the most unequal countries in the world with a huge divide between the poor and the rich. As such, the country faces several socio-economic challenges that have a bearing on reception and compliance to risk communication messages. According to the World Bank report "Overcoming Poverty and inequality in South Africa",[2] South Africa has an unemployment rate of 27.7% (2017) and poverty remains very high for a middle-income country. The labour market is split into two extreme job types. On the one hand, there are a small number of people in highly paid jobs in the formal sectors and corporations. On the other hand, there are the majority of the population in informal and poorly paid jobs. The latter include registered and non-registered migrants from neighbouring countries who reside in densely populated areas and informal settlements. There is a huge rural population.

The lockdown messages might have been clear for the authorities and the rich elites, but they did not make sense for the poor citizens. Several practical limitations undermined the government's strategy. The tough restrictions did not factor in the contextual realities in South Africa. In the major cities of Johannesburg, Pretoria, Cape Town, and Durban, there is a huge population of vagrants who obviously cannot be confirmed to any particular residence. In addition, one finds overcrowded informal settlements, squatter camps, and "occupied" buildings, home to thousands of poor locals, undocumented immigrants, and disabled persons who ordinarily live in extreme poverty and support themselves through begging, manual jobs, selling in the markets, or welfare. Given the socio-economic conditions in South Africa, where the majority have to leave their homes for their daily livelihood, it became clear that the public would not adhere to government measures.

In a country where many people stay in crowded and impoverished conditions, the government's blanket measures were simply impractical. How do you stay at home and self-isolate when you share your home and facilities like toilets and showers with many other residents, you get your running water from communal facilities, and your food resources do not last more than a day or so? In the absence of the most basic necessities, the poor in townships and informal settlements were most vulnerable to breaching the curfews. Social distancing went out of the window when residents left their homes in search of food. It became apparent that no amount of persuasion would dissuade people from leaving their homes and neither was the fear of COVID-19. It was a matter of survival. By staying at home, they faced imminent starvation.

Norway's *Dugnad* Moment

On Thursday 12 March 2020, the Norwegian government called for a press conference to announce what has been described as the strictest and most invasive measures Norway has ever had in peacetime. Prime Minister Erna Solberg was flanked by the Director of the Public Health Institute Camilla Stoltenberg, the Minister of Health and Care Services Bent Høie, and the Director of Health Bjørn Guldvog in announcing the wide-ranging lockdown measures in response to the COVID-19 situation. The following table provides a summary of the lockdown measures (Table 5.1).

Making people adhere to the lockdown message is not an easy task. In analysing the speeches, the persuasive narratives used in the communication of lockdown measures are examined. Elements drawn from Sellnow and Sellnow's (2011) IDEA (Internationalization, Distribution, Explanation, and Action) model for effective instructional and crisis messages are employed in the analysis. The narratives applied in government communications are explored.

Invitation til Dugnad: *Shared Responsibility and Togetherness*

The prime minister's shutdown speech emphasized shared responsibility and the need to stand together during the crisis. Solberg drew on the existing nationalistic cultural repertoire of the Norwegian concept of *dugnad* (Arora, Debesay, & Eslen-Ziya, 2022) and the collective spirit (*dugnadsånd*) it embraces (Nilsen & Skarpenes, 2022). The concept, *dugnad*, is a centuries-old tradition that relates to collective efforts and voluntary work done by individuals for the sake of the community. The word derives from the old Norse word *dugnaðr* meaning help, support or virtue, good quality (Moss & Sandbakken, 2021). It refers to a collective effort done in communities for such tasks as spring clearing, local sports clubs, housing associations, and helping neighbours in difficult situations.

Table 5.1 Norwegian government's COVID-19 (Office of the Prime Minister, 2020)

Recommendations	Mandatory
Hand hygiene and cough etiquette	Stay at home for those with infection symptoms
Work from home if possible	Home quarantine (i.e. returning residents, contact)
Use of public transport to be avoided	Home isolation (i.e. confirmed infections)
Limit leisure travel in Norway	Closure (i.e. educational institutions, restaurants)
No visits to health institutions	Cancelled/postponed (all events)
	International travel ban

The concept has a national cultural significance, described by others as distinctly Norwegian. In 1994, the word was selected as a national word because it says much about Norwegianness. As such, this is a word that has been in the Norwegian public discourse for centuries and hence has special significance. Most Norwegians relate to the concept of *dugnad*.

The government's crisis response narrative was anchored on a call for *dugnad*. In their research, Moss and Sandbakken (2021) found that from day one and throughout the COVID-19 period, the government used the term *dugnad* very actively in their press conferences. This narrative strategy echoes the WHO calls for a "whole of society" approach to combating COVID-19 infections. In trying to rally the whole of Norway to support the government lockdown measures, Solberg's speech appealed to this *dugnad* culture and spirit of the Norwegian people, inviting them to participate in what would be Norway's biggest *dugnad* to limit the damaging effects of COVID-19.

The speeches quoted in Table 5.2 illustrate the weight given to the *dugnad* as a cultural tool required to convince the inhabitants to accept the strong measures being implemented by the government, despite their stringent conditions and intrusions of individual freedoms. Moss and Sandbakken (2021) argue that using terminology familiar to the public appealed to a positive social identity as Norwegians working together for a shared goal. The message promoted togetherness in dealing with the issue at hand, just as the forefathers did in the past. In calling for the *dugnad*, the government was in a nuanced way instructing the inhabitants to stay at their homes, isolate themselves, or observe social distancing. Some scholars noted that the concept of *dugnad* was used to obscure the forced nature of the measures (Tjora, 2020). The strategy bore fruit, as evidenced by the degree of adherence to lockdown measures in Norway. As Nilsen and Skarpenes (2022) conclude, by appealing to the people's sense of collective effort Norwegian leaders successfully managed to co-ordinate the actions of the population and controlled the outbreak (Table 5.3).

The messages were disseminated during a press conference, which was also streamed on other media platforms, and was reported widely through media such as the radio and newspapers.

Trust and Solidarity

Trust is another factor that the Norwegian government exploited in its lockdown communication. In a press conference held on the 18 March 2020, Prime Minister Erna Solberg emphasized the significance of trust in Norwegian society. She pointed to the magnitude of the crisis faced by the country and its citizens – and remarked that no one in her generation has experienced that the country has such great challenges as "we are facing together now". She reminds the people that Norway has gone through difficult times before but "we will make it this time too. Together", because the country has trust as its strongest weapon. Because

Table 5.2 The Norwegian "dugnad" moment

The "dugnad" narrative		
Health Minister Bent Høie	Debate post in the VG 11 March 2020	Call for *dugnad* (VG).[a] "Now we need *dugnad* in the Norwegian society". "All sectors must contribute to the *dugnad*" "We take measures to prevent the spread of infection and ensure that the seriously ill receive healthcare. But the whole of society must participate in the work against the coronavirus. Each one of us has an important task".
Prime Minister Erna Solberg	Government Press Conference 12 March 2020	"We know that the virus infects when people meet or are close to each other, therefore it is very crucial that all the nation's citizens participate in a *dugnad* to slow down the infection". "In Norway we stand together when it counts. We mobilize to *dugnad* and collaboration in small and larger communities, and this is more important now than ever before".
Health Minister Bent Høie	Government Press Conference 12 March 2020	"These measures are some of the strictest that we have in our toolbox and we do this in the hope to prevent the spread of the virus". "These measures will be experienced as a burden for many and will have a big consequence for Norwegian society. But this is a *dugnad* that we need to take as a community and on behalf of the community".
Health Minister Bent Høie	13 March 2020	"I am incredibly grateful for the way these measures that we presented yesterday have been received". "My experience is that the whole population now are on board for the good *dugnad*".
Health Minister Bent Høie	20 March 2020	"It may be that this *dugnad* will last longer than we hope and want".

[a] Debate post in VG by Bent Høie https://www.vg.no/nyheter/meninger/i/EWnBO3/innkalling-til-dugnad (Accessed 14.02.2023).

people trust each other and trust in the leadership, the country will prevail over the crisis. She reassures the population that the country's leadership is united (Table 5.4):

The government, the Stortinget (parliament) and the whole of political Norway are doing everything in their power to get us safely through this difficult period. Our common desire to do the best for everyone who lives in Norway will always be greater than our disagreements".[3]

Table 5.3 Analysis of the lockdown press conference 12 March using the IDEA model

IDEA Element	
Internalization	The coronavirus is spreading fast.
	The scenario shows that many will die in Norway.
	The everyday life of many will be turned upside down.
Explanation	We are entering a difficult time for Norway and the world.
	Norway is being put to the test, both as a society and as individuals.
Action	We all must protect ourselves in order to protect others.
	We stand together in this period, not with hugs and handshakes, but to keep our distance.
	This requires a lot from each of us, we should care for and help each other. We have managed before and I am sure we will manage.
	We should do this in solidarity with the elderly and the chronically sick and others that are especially exposed to developing a serious illness.

Table 5.4 Trust as a weapon

Date		
15 March 2020	Minister of Justice Monica Mæland	"There are not many countries in the world where the authorities can introduce the most intrusive rules of peacetime, with a population that responds by saying 'yes, we will partake in this'".
18 March 2020	Prime Minister Erna Solberg	"The generations before us have created a society where we have trust in, and respect for, each other".
		"When terror and accidents have befallen us, we have gone through it together. When freedom has been threatened, Norwegians have given everything for each other".
		"This has given our country an advantage that is more powerful than any weapon, and more valuable than any oil fund: Namely, that *we trust each other*".
		"It is this trust that will carry us through the crisis we are now facing".
		"Without the high level of trust between citizens and the authorities, we could never have got the whole of Norway involved in the effort to fight the Coronavirus".
		"In times of crisis, we understand how dependent we are on each other. What brings us together is more important than what divides us".
19 March 2020	Justice Minister Monica Mæland	"… there is something special about Norway. The trust we have in each other is more powerful than any weapon and more valuable than any oil fund".

The above analysis shows that the Norwegian government's outbreak communication benefited from the pre-existing cultural norms and the higher levels of trust and social capital in the country. The political leadership anchored their lockdown messages on the centuries-old *dugnad* culture, which resonated well with the majority of the population. Expression of shared responsibility distributed the societal risk to everyone in a relatively homogenous country. The higher level of trust between the citizens and the authorities created a conducive context that created positive effects for adherence to lockdown messages. As Johnsson et al. (2023) noted in their research on the pandemic communication in the Scandinavian countries, the high levels of trust provided a good starting point for successful crisis communication when the COVID-19 pandemic hit.

Conclusion – "One-Size Does Not Fit All"

The case studies discussed in this chapter underlie the fundamental importance of communication context in shaping the reception and outcomes of the lockdown messages. Similar messages delivered in different contexts can have different responses from the audience in terms of adherence and compliance. Responses to the declaration of the coronavirus as a pandemic have been fragmented with countries taking their own strategies, ranging from strict lockdowns to no lockdowns. As noted in the South African case study, the full lockdown strategy was the least pragmatic approach given the socio-economic conditions in the country. Even though the *thuma mina* messages were quite appealing to the public, a full lockdown was not feasible due to other socio-economic factors. Other factors such as the lower levels of institutional trust contributed to non-compliance with lockdown measures. This led the South African government to resort to military enforcement of the lockdown. In the Norwegian case study, the *dugnad* lockdown messages were appealing to the public and were equally backed by a strong social welfare culture and high trust levels that created positive effects for the messages. The cases illustrate that "one-size-fits-all" public health strategy response to the coronavirus outbreak is not advisable due to local nuances. Messages should ideally be anchored on local conditionalities.

Notes

1 Ramaphosa, C. 2020. "'The most definitive Thuma Mina moment' for SA: Ramaphosa's plan for Covid-19" (Available at https://www.news24.com/SouthAfrica/News/read-in-full-the-most-definitive-thuma-mina-moment-for-sa-ramaphosas-plan-for-covid-19-20200315, Accessed 25.10.2022).
2 https://documents1.worldbank.org/curated/en/530481521735906534/pdf/Overcoming-Poverty-and-Inequality-in-South-Africa-An-Assessment-of-Drivers-Constraints-and-Opportunities.pdf (Accessed 19.10.2022).
3 https://www.aftenposten.no/norge/i/K3957e/statsminister-erna-solbergs-tale-til-folket-i-forbindelse-med-koronakrisen (Accessed 14.02.2023).

References

Arora, S., Debesay, J., & Eslen-Ziya, H. (2022). Persuasive narrative during the COVID-19 pandemic: Norwegian Prime Minister Erna Solberg's posts on Facebook. *Humanities and Social Sciences Communications, 9*(1), 35. doi:10.1057/s41599-022-01051-5

Atkin, C. (2001). Theory and principles of media health campaigns. In R. Rice & C. Atkin (Eds.), *Public Communication Campaigns* (3 ed.) (pp. 49–68). London: Sage Publications.

Bester, P., Els, S., & Olivier, L. (2020). Deployment of the South African national defence force for COVID-19: A case study on governance. *AJPSDG, 3*(1), 106–133.

Buchholz, K. (2020). What share of the world population is already on Covid-19 lockdowns? Retrieved from https://www.statista.com/chart/21240/enforced-covid-19-lockdowns-by-people-affected-per-country/

Haider, N., Osman, A. Y., Gadzekpo, A., Akipede, G. O., Asogun, D., Ansumana, R., . . . McCoy, D. (2020). Lockdown measures in response to COVID-19 in nine sub-Saharan African countries. *BMJ Global Health, 5*(10), e003319. Doi:10.1136/bmjgh-2020-003319

Johnsson, B., Ihlen, Ø., Lindholm, J., & Blach-Ørsten, M. (2023). Introduction: Communicating a pandemic in the Nordic countries. In B. Johnsson, Ø. Ihlen, J. Lindholm, & M. Blach-Ørsten (Eds.), *Communicating a Pandemic: Crisis Management and Covid-19 in the Nordic Countries* (pp. 11–30). Gothenburg, Sweden: Nordicom.

Maluleke, T. (2018) Op-Ed: The deep roots of Ramaphosa's 'Thuma Mina'. South Africa. *Daily Maverick.* https://www.dailymaverick.co.za/article/2018-02-22-op-ed-the-deep-roots-of-ramaphosas-thuma-mina/ (Accessed 25.10.2022).

Mawere, T. (2020). Uniting against the common enemy: Covid-19 and South Africa's militarised nationhood. Retrieved from https://www.csagup.org/2020/04/15/uniting-against-the-common-enemy-covid-19-and-south-africas-militarised-nationhood/

Migliaccio, M., Buono, A., Maltese, I., & Migliaccio, M. (2021). The 2020 Italian spring lockdown: A multidisciplinary analysis over the Milan urban area. *World, 2*(3), 391–414.

Moss, S. M., & Sandbakken, E. M. (2021). "Everybody Needs to do their part, so we can get this under control." Reactions to the Norwegian Government Meta-Narratives on COVID-19 measures. *Political Psychology, 42*(5), 881–898. doi: 10.1111/pops.12727

Nilsen, A. C. E., & Skarpenes, O. (2022). Coping with COVID-19. Dugnad: A case of the moral premise of the Norwegian welfare state. *International Journal of Sociology and Social Policy, 42*(3/4), 262–275. doi:10.1108/IJSSP-07-2020-0263

Office of the Prime Minister. (2020). Omfattende tiltak for å bekjempe koronaviruset [Press release]. Retrieved from https://www.regjeringen.no/no/dokumentarkiv/regjeringen-solberg/aktuelt-regjeringen-solberg/smk/pressemeldinger/2020/nye-tiltak/id2693327/

Rothstein, M. A., Alcalde, M. G., Elster, N. R., Majumder, M. A., Palmer, L., & Stone, T. (2003). Quarantine and isolation: Lessons learned from SARS, a report to the Centers for Disease Control and Prevention. Atlanta, GA: CDC. Retrieved https://stacks.cdc.gov/view/cdc/11429 (Accessed 21.06.2023).

Salmon, C. T., & Atkin, C. (2003). Using media campaigns for health promotion. In T. L. Thompson, A. M. Dorsey, K. Miller, & R. Parrott (Eds.), *Handbook of Health Communication* (pp. 449–472). London: Lawrence Erlbaum Associates.

Seekings, J., & Nattrass, N. (2020). Covid vs. democracy: South Africa's Lockdown Misfire. *Journal of Democracy, 31*(4), 106–121.

Sellnow, T. L., & Sellnow, D. D. (2011). *Messages Matter: Crisis Communication Strategies for Encouraging Self-Protection.* Little Rock, AR: Center for Toxicology and Environmental Health.

Smart, B. T. H., Broadbent, A., & Combrink, H. (2020). Lockdown didnt work in South Africa: Why it shouldn't happen again. *Prevention Web.* Retrieved from https://www.preventionweb.net/news/lockdown-didnt-work-south-africa-why-it-shouldnt-happen-again

Tjora, A. (2020). Tillitsfull dugnad eller instruert solidaritet, Chronicle. *Universitetsavisa.* Retrieved from https://www.universitetsavisa.no/koronavirus-ytring/tillitsfull-dugnad-eller-instruert-solidaritet/111642

Tognotti, E. (2013). Lessons from the history of quarantine, from plague to influenza A. *Emerging Infectious Disease, 19*(2), 254–259. doi:10.3201/eid1902.120312

WHO. (2021). Considerations for quarantine of contacts of COVID-19 cases: Interim guidance, 25 June 2021. Retrieved from Geneva: https://apps.who.int/iris/handle/10665/342004

6 Communicating Uncertainty

Introduction

Much of the literature on crisis communication emphasizes the need to communicate quickly when responding to an emergency. In public health crises, rapid dissemination of information about the disease and the recommended protective measures is essential to minimize or prevent the spread of the disease and to avert health risks. The crisis communication discipline offers numerous pieces of advice on what, how, and when to communicate during a crisis. However, this presumes that there is certainty in the negative outcomes of the crisis. Yet in most crises, the knowledge base required for guiding meaningful communication is lacking, inadequate, or uncertain. In any crisis, uncertainty is ever-present, whether we like it or not. Many definitions of crisis and crisis communication acknowledge the presence of uncertainty (Coombs, 2019; Seeger, 2006). "Risks are always associated with some level of uncertainty, and crises, are, by definition, high-uncertainty events, where information is often not immediately available" (Seeger, 2006, pp. 239–240). A crisis like a health pandemic involves various degrees of uncertainty, be it scientific facts about the disease, models for forecasting its spreading, and estimates of mortality rates. Uncertainty is a crucial element of any risk assessment, and consequently, it poses many challenges to communication. Uncertainty in the degree of risk in health is a major challenge for risk and crisis communication. How should public health authorities communicate uncertainties? Or as Baker and Hernandez (2017) pose, how do you communicate with audiences when the nature of the bad news is uncertain and open to multiple interpretations? What are the positive and negative effects associated with their choices? This uncertainty must be communicated efficiently, if the relevant authorities and the public are to make sound conclusions about the imminent threat of the pandemic. How health authorities communicate uncertainty affects public trust and has an impact on the acceptance or non-acceptance of the messages. This chapter examines the issue of uncertainty and the challenges of communicating uncertainty during a pandemic. It argues that if uncertainty is not adequately communicated, it can

DOI: 10.4324/9781003401827-6

hamper decision-making, undermine trust in communicators and messages, and consequently affect the public's behavioural response to the pandemic. It argues that trust is fundamental to the effectiveness of uncertainty messages.

Defining Uncertainty

The *Cambridge Dictionary* defines uncertainty as "a situation in which something is not known, or something that is not known or certain".[1] The *Merriam-Webster* dictionary defines uncertainty as "the quality and state of being uncertain". It refers to the state of being in doubt, being unsure, and not fully knowing. The concept of "uncertainty" is widely used in crisis communication research, especially in the field of health communication. Brashers (2001, p. 478) argues that "uncertainty exists when details of situations are ambiguous, complex, unpredictable, or probabilistic; when information is unavailable or inconsistent; and when people feel insecure about their state of knowledge or the state of knowledge in general". Coombs (2015, p. 112) argues that uncertainty is the amount of ambiguity associated with a problem, and the larger the amount of ambiguity surrounding a crisis, the greater the uncertainty. Most crises have elements of uncertainty in addition to being information-power and knowledge-poor situations.

Sources of Uncertainty in COVID-19

The imprecise nature of disease science contributes to uncertainty. Uncertainty is the defining feature of public health crisis, and as Han et al. (2011) correctly indicate, "uncertainty pervades and motives every activity related to health care". In describing uncertainty in medical practice, Eddy (1984) notes that:

> uncertainty creeps into medical practice through every pore. Whether a physician is defining a disease, making a diagnosis, selecting a procedure, observing outcomes, assessing probabilities, assigning preferences, or putting it all together, he (or she) is walking on very slippery terrain.

Not surprisingly, the COVID-19 disease was associated with uncertainty, be it questions about its aetiology (i.e. issues related to its causes and manifestations) and management. Koffman et al. (2020) use the phrase "known – unknowns" and "unknown – unknowns" to describe various uncertainties surrounding COVID-19. They identify four sets of uncertainties: (1) disease uncertainties, (2) health system uncertainties, (3) health professional uncertainties, and (4) patient- and family centred uncertainties. The coronavirus progressed into a pandemic within a context characterized by high levels of disease uncertainties. There was uncertainty in disease identification (is there a risk?) and another uncertainty in risk characterization (how high is the risk?).

Koffman et al. (2020) note that even when millions of confirmed cases of COVID-19 had been reported in many countries across the world (of whom millions have died), there was still much which was still unknown about the disease. It was not yet known why some individuals and groups were more affected than others. There was still confusion about the uncertain denominator making true mortality figures hard to quantify, compounded by the unknown prevalence of asymptomatic infection. As such, the COVID-19 pandemic presented unprecedented uncertainty in terms of how healthcare should respond to the crisis (ibid.). Another form of uncertainty surrounded the testing procedures and how heath care should handle patients who had tested positive for COVID-19. This uncertainty included basic hospital resources, medication, and the highly publicized provision of personal protective equipment (Koffman et al., 2020). Different facets of COVID-19 embodied various degrees of uncertainty.

There are many sources of uncertainty, but these can be put into two broad categories: scientific uncertainty and epistemic uncertainty. Scientific uncertainty refers to variations in quantitative measurements. No measurement can be completely accurate and errors in data are imminent. Scientific findings are not definitive and hence there is no 100 per cent certainty. New evidence or the addition of new variables can nullify previous findings and predictions. In science, research is an ongoing practice. Scientific uncertainty means different things in different fields like natural sciences, social sciences, and the humanities (Landström, Hauxwell-Baldwin, Lorenzoni, & Rogers-Hayden, 2015). These interpretations have different implications for decision-making and communication. It is no wonder that scientific uncertainty is often at the centre of public controversies. Lack of certainty often causes problems when decisions and actions are taken. Scientific uncertainty plays a crucial role in the formulation of public policy. Decision-makers in society use scientific inputs when devising new policies.

Epistemic uncertainty refers to a lack of knowledge or information. One of the most recurrent themes in most crisis communication literature is the *lack of knowledge* (Rogers, Amlôt, Rubin, Wessely, & Krieger, 2007). Lack of knowledge is a defining characteristic of any disease outbreak, simply because one does not have much knowledge about the nature of an outbreak, how it will spread, and how the infected will react to it. The models used by epidemiologists to forecast the path of the COVID-19 pandemic have their advantages and limitations. Emerging infectious diseases are characterized by the scarcity of knowledge and a higher prevalence of uncertainty, simply because they are unknown and unpredictable. Emerging infectious diseases are often shrouded with several uncertainties, for example, the likelihood of something happening according to a particular forecast or issues of "uncertainty about the uncertainty" also referred to as epistemic uncertainty. We can never be completely certain about the trajectory of diseases. There will always be uncertainty around them. For example, mutations in viruses occur frequently and they sometimes change the characteristics of the disease, with positive or negative public health implications.

When the coronavirus outbreak was first reported in China, no one could have predicted that it would escalate into a full pandemic. As the WHO (World Health Organization) admitted, this was the first pandemic caused by a coronavirus. The source of the uncertainty in this pandemic was the lack of enough expert knowledge about the virus. The experts did not have all the information about the nature of the virus; hence the uncertainty about the potential seriousness of the threat and actions that should be taken by individuals and governments. As an unfolding risk still under study, there were no conclusive results and hard facts about the virus to inform decision-making. Its development was a matter of probabilities.

The most contestable aspect of COVID-19 has been the degree of scientific uncertainty and the consequent justifications for measures and restrictions. Lack of conclusive knowledge, that is, scientifically proven data, contradictory findings, and ambiguity (contractions between scientists) undermined the justifications for stringent measures and restrictions. If authorities do not possess conclusive data about a phenomenon, then they cannot use it as a justification for introducing intrusive measures. Contradictory data is one of the sources of uncertainty identified by Liu et al. (2016) in their review of knowledge gaps in communicating crisis uncertainty, in addition to the lack of knowledge and ambiguity that arises when there are contradictions between experts. COVID-19 was imbued in uncertainty. As such, there were grounds for multiple interpretations of the unfolding virus pandemic.

Theories on Communication and Uncertainty

Health contexts and crises are characterized by the pervasiveness of uncertainty. Researchers have pondered over the issue of uncertainty and how best one can communicate effectively in times of uncertainty (Liu et al., 2016). Outside the field of crisis communication research approaches such as the uncertainty reduction theory (Berger & Calabrese, 1975) and uncertainty management theory (Brashers, 2001) are some of the most prominent theories. The uncertainty reduction theory assumes that humans are motivated to decrease uncertainty about themselves and others. Uncertainty is viewed as negative and something that needs to be mitigated. The uncertainty management theory assumes that people experience uncertainty differently and not only in a negative way, but can be positive, neutral, or negative. The theory propose that people may want to reduce, maintain, or even increase their uncertainty, depending on their appraisals of and emotional responses to experiences characterized by uncertainty (Babrow & Stone, 2021). For example, individuals who experience uncertainty that causes distress might try to reduce that uncertainty. People might engage in information seeking or information avoidance to sustain a desired level of uncertainty or certainty (ibid.). Bradac (2006) argues that people can seek information to strategically increase (rather than reduce) uncertainty. Information seeking and avoiding is seen as a communication means of managing uncertainty (Babrow & Stone, 2021).

To address the challenges of uncertainty, van der Bles et al. (2019) suggest a framework for communicating epistemic uncertainty based on Harold Lasswell's model of communication. This classical model, formulated by Harold Lasswell in 1948, describes an act of communication by defining who (the communicator) says what (message) in which channel (the medium) to whom (receiver) and with what effect. Van der Bles et al. revisit this classical model and try to address questions like "who communicates what, in what form, to whom, and to what effect" while acknowledging the relevant context as part of the characteristics of the audience.

The Communicator

The first factor in Han et al.'s framework is to examine the communicator of uncertainty. The communicator's characteristics have a bearing on the reception of the messages. The research underlines the importance of identifying the communicator of uncertainty. In health pandemics, there are two groups of communicators. The first group includes the people assessing uncertainty (e.g. various scientific experts such as epidemiologist and statistical organizations). According to van der Bles et al., these are the real owners of uncertainty. The second group includes communication practitioners – those that do the communication (e.g. communication professionals, journalists, and those acting on behalf of institutions). It is important to identify who is communicating uncertainty, as people assessing and communicating are many and varied. Communicators might also have different intentions as to what they want to achieve for their audiences. Several factors influence the choice of communication form and the effects of communication.

In the US, for example, one of the main obstacles in the communication of uncertainty was the lack of a unified front by the public authorities. An article by *Scientific American* (2021)[2] aptly describes what went wrong with the American response to the COVID-19 pandemic, namely the sidelining of experts, the people whom van der Bles et al. (2019) describe as the real owners of uncertainty. "During the pandemic's crucial early days and weeks, then President Donald Trump and other public figures actively underplayed the threat of the virus. Trump dismissed it as no worse than the flu and said the pandemic would be over by Easter" (*Scientific American*). Senior public figures in the Trump administration did not take the threat seriously. Lewis (ibid.) notes that when a spokesperson for the US Centers for Disease Control and Prevention (CDC) acknowledged that the threat of coronavirus could be severe, the agency was quickly sidelined – and Trump himself became the government's main conduit for COVID-19 updates:

> This muzzling of the CDC and top government health experts made it hard for them to communicate accurate and lifesaving scientific information to the public.
>
> (*Scientific American*, 11 March 2021)

In the US case, communication of scientific uncertainty floundered due to disregard for expertise. In contrast, in Sweden, it was not the politicians, but the Public Health Agency with state epidemiologist Anders Tegnell in charge of communicating uncertainty. Therefore, the task of communicating scientific uncertainty was left to public health experts, the real owners of uncertainty.

Several factors impact on the communication of uncertainty. Liu et al. (2016) identify three key variables related to uncertainty communication: trust, fear, and the information source. On the variable of trust, Liu et al. (2016) argue that trust and uncertainty interact in two main ways: first, the impact of the public trust in the communicator on their acceptable of uncertainty; and second, the impact of the communicator's admission of uncertainty on the public's trust in the communicator (p. 481). The main argument raised is that the more the public trust their government or the communicating official, the better they can handle fear in uncertain situations. A lack of trust in the communicator would have adverse effects on the messages and the desired behavioural changes. The Ebola crisis in West Africa provides succinct evidence of what happens when local people do not trust their public officials and do not feel obliged to follow the required recommendations. Why should we trust you when you don't even care about us? Why should we listen to you when you are also unsure? These are some of the comments from the public when governments in Africa sought to control the COVID-19 pandemic in their neighbourhoods. Distrust in the communicator can exacerbate the crisis.

The Message

The second factor in Han et al.'s framework addresses *what* is being communicated. How should uncertainty be communicated in the messages? Van der Bles et al. identify four sub-factors that should be considered in examining what is communicated, that is, the object about which there is uncertainty (e.g. facts and statistics on the coronavirus); the source of uncertainty (such as the lack of knowledge on the coronavirus); the level of uncertainty (e.g. lack of confidence in the underlying science concerning the epidemic); and finally, the magnitude of the uncertainty, the level and the magnitude of uncertainty. The messages must be clear about the source and magnitude of uncertainty. For example, when presenting COVID-19 statistics, it is also important to communicate how they are derived and the possibilities of errors in the measurements. Lack of openness (on uncertainty) in statistics saw public authorities being questioned or challenged by the members of the public who were quite aware of the inadequacies in statistical information. In South Africa, for example, a study showed that there was about three times the number of excess deaths from natural causes during 2020 and 2021 than the reported COVID-19 deaths.[3] This means that more people may have died of COVID-19 than reported by the authorities. How certain you are about something (e.g. 10%, 50%, or 90% certain) is important for decision-making by those targeted by the message.

The Audience

The third factor in the Han et al.'s model is the form of communication in which uncertainty is communicated to the public. It can be through the presentation of probabilities, visualization, and the medium used in the communication. The third factor focuses on the audiences, that is, to whom uncertainty is communicated. The characteristics of the audiences (their literacy, expertise, and knowledge of the field), the nature of the relationship between the communicator and the audience (e.g. trust or distrust between the communicator and the audience), and the relationship between the audience and what is being communicated is crucial for the communication of uncertainty. Sometimes, the topic of what is being communicated, for example, restrictions on people's movements, is highly contested or triggers a lot of emotions. Finally, the last factors pertain to the effect of the communication on the audience's cognition, emotion, trust and behaviour, and decision-making.

Communicating Uncertainty During the Pandemic

Public health crises such as the COVID-19 pandemic pose difficult communication challenges, due in large part to the substantial scientific uncertainty surrounding the nature and management of all new and emerging health threats (P. Han et al., 2021). Uncertainty is a central trait of a public health crisis. Lack of facts about a new disease outbreak hampers decision-making and political leadership in public health emergencies. Public health officials face challenges in communicating with the public about emerging diseases due to epistemic uncertainty. As Van der Bles et al. (2019) note, "all knowledge on which decisions and policies are based – from medical evidence to government statistics – are shrouded with epistemic uncertainty of different types and degrees" (p. 2) (van der Bles et al., 2019). Han et al. (2021) note that uncertainty caused by a lack of reliability, credibility, or adequacy of risk information produces a set of cognitive, emotional, and behavioural responses. These responses include heightened risk perceptions, pessimistic appraisals of risk-reducing actions, fear and anxiety, and avoidance of decision-making (p. 2).

Communicating uncertainty is fundamental to any response to a health pandemic because over- or under-communicating uncertainty can impact negatively on the crisis. In an era of contested expertise, many shy away from openly communicating their uncertainty about what they know, fearful of their audience's reaction (van der Bles et al., 2019). In an article "Communicating Uncertainty: Fulfilling the Duty to Inform",[4] Fischhoff (2012) notes that scientists are often hesitant to share their uncertainty with decision-makers who need to know it. There is an assumption among many scientists and policymakers that communicating uncertainty might have negative consequences, such as signalling incompetence, encouraging critics, and decreasing trust (Fischhoff, 2012). However, other researchers argue that on the contrary, "communicating uncertainty can increase, rather than decrease, an individual's confidence and trust in information when they expect such uncertainty to exist" (P. Han et al., 2021, p. 2).

"A critical challenge in communicating the results of scientific research arises when those results contain a great deal of uncertainty" (Patt, 2009). Results from a scientific study can be invalidated in subsequent studies. Fleerackers et al. (2022) investigated the surge in the use of COVID-19-related preprints by media outlets, despite the scientific uncertainty inherent in them. Preprints are generally recognized by the scientific community as unvalidated and uncertain science. Sharing research findings from these sources can be misleading to the public. Fleerackers et al. (2022) note, for example, a case of a widely circulated COVID-19 preprint linking the SARS-CoV-2 spike protein to HIV-1 glycoproteins. The paper was later withdrawn by the authors following criticism from other scientists. The uncertainty in research findings presents challenges to the journalists wanting to inform the public. Sometimes, journalists do ignore these uncertainties when sharing research findings.

Scientists face the challenges of communicating uncertainty to other decision-makers. Sometimes, decision-makers do not have complete knowledge about the disease to meet the public information needs and at the same time, they cannot afford the luxury of waiting too long in answering the questions, lest that void is filled by misinformation. Citing the case of the H1N1 pandemic, Fogarty et al. (2011) note that "statements intended to create awareness and convey the seriousness of infectious disease threats can draw accusations of scaremongering, while officials can be accused of complacency if such statements are not made" (p.1). This is a real dilemma which needs a proper balancing act, with the government balancing all the competing priorities and reducing fear. As Ndlela (2019) argues, in emergency cases, a timely decision based on some information is better than a delayed decision with complete information.

What Are the Best Ways to Communicate Uncertainty?

Averting the challenges of communicating scientific uncertainty has been a central focus for public health organizations. The Crisis and Emergency Risk Communication (CERC)[5] issued by the US CDC takes special note of the inherent challenges. It notes that there are often more questions than answers during a crisis, especially in the beginning, and this uncertainty will challenge even the greatest communicator. CERC recommends that communicators should acknowledge uncertainty and also empathize with the audience's uncertainty. Communicators should tell their audiences:

- What is known
- What is not known
- What is done to reduce the uncertainty

CERC further warns against promoting excess certainty about future outcomes that cannot be controlled. Uncertainty can have negative psychological effects such as heightening perceptions of risk and promoting fear, panic, anxiety, emotional distress, and feelings of hopelessness and helplessness, which can prevent people from taking action (CERC)[6].

Given the inevitability of uncertainty in the public health crisis, global health organizations like the WHO (2020) have outlined a set of recommendations. These are:

- Be transparent
- Explicitly communicate information about uncertainty
- Maintain consistency over time
- Maintain consistency in communication among partners
- Communicate action

Researchers like Rogers et al. (2007) conclude that it is better for officials to admit uncertainty than to present information or assurances as certain and be proven wrong later. WHO recommends that "communication by authorities to the public should include explicit information about uncertainties associated with risks, events and interventions, and indicate what is known and not known at a given time" (WHO, 2017).

Conclusion

Uncertainty is pervasive in a public health crisis and communicators need to navigate the challenges of communicating to the public even when some information is not complete or uncertain. Understanding the context and the audience is vital in the communication of uncertainty. Uncertainty has many dimensions and many sources, and as such, individuals react differently to the stimulus. Some audiences have a greater tolerance for uncertainty, while others have a lower threshold. Communicating uncertainty strengthens confidence in some, but too much uncertainty can impact the public negatively. Admitting that the health experts are uncertain can be interpreted negatively – that they don't know what they are talking about and hence their policies and measures can consequently be ignored. In the early phases of the coronavirus pandemic, an inadequate understanding of the virus and its trajectory made risk and crisis communication challenging. This challenge underlies the need for an effective and contextualized message.

Notes

1 2018 Cambridge dictionary. Cambridge: Cambridge University Press.
2 https://www.scientificamerican.com/article/how-the-u-s-pandemic-response-went-wrong-and-what-went-right-during-a-year-of-covid/ (Accessed 09.09.2020).
3 https://www.news.uct.ac.za/images/userfiles/downloads/media/2022_06_09_ExcessNaturalDeaths.pdf (Accessed 18.04.2023).
4 Communicating Uncertainty: Fulfilling the Duty to Inform https://issues.org/fischhoff/ (Accessed 23.02.2021).
5 https://emergency.cdc.gov/cerc/ppt/CERC_Psychology_of_a_Crisis.pdf (Accessed 09.09.2021).
6 https://emergency.cdc.gov/cerc/ppt/CERC_Psychology_of_a_Crisis.pdf (Accessed 09.09.21).

References

Babrow, A. S., & Stone, A. M. (2021). Theories of communication and uncertainty as a foundation for future research on nursing practice. *Nursing Communication, 1*(1), 1–22.

Baker, S., & Hernandez, M. (2017). Communicating with stakeholders when bad news is uncertain. *International Journal of Public Leadership, 13*(2), 85–97. doi:10.1108/IJPL-11-2016-0051

Berger, C. R., & Calabrese, R. J. (1975). Some explorations in initial interaction and beyond: Toward a Developmental theory of interpersonal communication. *Human Communication Research, 1*(2), 99–112. https://doi.org/10.1111/j.1468-2958.1975.tb00258.x

Bradac, J. J. (2006). Theory comparison: Uncertainty Reduction, problematic integration, uncertainty management, and other curious constructs. *Journal of Communication, 51*(3), 456–476. doi:10.1111/j.1460-2466.2001.tb02891.x %J Journal of Communication

Brashers, D. E. (2001). Communication and uncertainty management. *Journal of Communication, 51*(3), 477–497.

Coombs, W. T. (2015). *Ongoing Crisis Communication: Planning, Managing, and Responding* (4 ed.). Los Angeles, CA: Sage.

Coombs, W. T. (2019). *Ongoing Crisis Communication. Planning, Managing, and Responding* (5 ed.). Los Angeles, CA: Sage.

Eddy, D. M. (1984). Variations in physician practice: The role of uncertainty. *Health Affairs (Millwood), 3*(2), 74–89. doi:10.1377/hlthaff.3.2.74

Fischhoff, B. (2012). Communicating uncertainty: Fulfilling the duty to inform. *Issues in Science and Technology, 28*, 63–70.

Fleerackers, A., Riedlinger, M., Moorhead, L., Ahmed, R., & Alperin, J. P. (2022). Communicating scientific uncertainty in an age of COVID-19: An Investigation into the use of preprints by digital media outlets. *Health Communication, 37*(6), 726–738. doi:10.1080/10410236.2020.1864892

Fogarty, A. S., Holland, K., Imison, M., Blood, R. W., Chapman, S., & Holding, S. (2011). Communicating uncertainty - how Australian television reported H1N1 risk in 2009: A content analysis. *BMC Public Health, 11*(1), 181. doi:10.1186/1471-2458-11-181

Han, P. K. J., Klein, W. M. P., & Arora, N. K. (2011). Varieties of uncertainty in health care: A conceptual taxonomy. *Medical Decision Making: An International Journal of the Society for Medical Decision Making, 31*(6), 828–838. doi:10.1177/0272989x11393976

Han, P., Scharnetzki, E., Scherer, A., Thorpe, A., Lary, C., Waterston, L., . . . Dieckmann, N. (2021). Communicating scientific uncertainty about the COVID-19 Pandemic: Online experimental study of an uncertainty-normalizing strategy. *Journal of Medical Internet Research, 23*(4), 1–12. doi:10.2196/27832

Koffman, J., Gross, J., Etkind, S. N., & Selman, L. (2020). Uncertainty and COVID-19: How are we to respond? *Journal of the Royal Society of Medicine, 113*(6), 211–216. doi:10.1177/0141076820930665

Landström, C., Hauxwell-Baldwin, R., Lorenzoni, I., & Rogers-Hayden, T. (2015). The (mis)understanding of scientific uncertainty? How experts view policy-makers, the media and publics. *Science as Culture, 24*(3), 276–298. doi:10.1080/09505431.2014.992333

Liu, B. F., Bartz, L., & Duke, N. (2016). Communicating crisis uncertainty: A review of the knowledge gaps. *Public Relations Review, 42*(3), 479–487. doi:10.1016/j.pubrev.2016.03.003

Patt, A. (2009). Communicating uncertainty to policy makers. In L. M. & M. J. (Eds.), *Uncertainties in Environmental Modelling and Consequences for Policy Making* (pp. 231–251). Dordrecht: Springer.

Rogers, M. B., Amlôt, R., Rubin, G. J., Wessely, S., & Krieger, K. (2007). Mediating the social and psychological impacts of terrorist attacks: The role of risk perception and risk communication. *International Review of Psychiatry, 19*(3), 279–288. doi:10.1080/09540260701349373

Seeger, M. W. (2006). Best practices in crisis communication: An expert panel process. *Journal of Applied Communication Research, 34*(3), 232–244. doi:10.1080/00909880600769944

van der Bles, A. M., van der Linden, S., Freeman, A. L. J., Mitchell, J., Galvao, A. B., Zaval, L., & Spiegelhalter, D. J. (2019). Communicating uncertainty about facts, numbers and science. *Royal Society Open Science, 6*(5). doi:10.1098/rsos.181870

WHO. (2017). Communicating risk in public health emergencies: A WHO guideline for emergency risk communication (ERC) policy and practice. https://apps.who.int/iris/bitstream/handle/10665/259807/9789241550208-eng.pdf

7   Risk Messages, Form, and Context

Introduction

The messages are central to any health communication. In epidemics and pandemics, effective communication of risk messages is essential for mitigating loss of life. Risk messages enable people to make informed decisions about how they can protect their health and their lives. During a pandemic, individuals need to understand the risk they face and how best they can protect themselves from infection. The decision-making process is best served when the risk is clearly communicated, understood, and acted upon through a change of behaviour. The goal of risk and crisis communication during a pandemic is to change behaviour. Messages seek to inform and educate the target population on what they should do during the crisis. They also provide compelling evidence and facts on why people need to act as told. Finally, they provide specific guidelines, tools, and skills to guide the actions. Effective risk communication educates the public about health risks, boosts awareness, and promotes risk-reducing behaviours necessary for mitigating and controlling the pandemic. Morgan and Lave (1990) state that risk messages must be understood by the recipients and their impacts and effectiveness must be understood by the communicator. Compliance and non-compliance with the messages have consequences for individuals and society at large. In crisis and emergency risk communication, the audience interacts with the messages they receive. They make evaluations of the source of the messages and the attributes of the sender.

The coronavirus pandemic once again highlighted the importance of health messages and the complexities in crafting and presenting the content of the message in a highly complex, uncertain, and dynamic crisis context. Health authorities and other crisis leaders created a plethora of messages daily in their quest to manage the pandemic and its other related crises. This chapter explores the inherent challenges of formulating and presenting messages during a pandemic. It looks at the critical aspect of risk communication messages, the strategies, purposes, and contexts. The fundamental assumption of this chapter is that people can be hurt if messages are poorly formulated and presented.

DOI: 10.4324/9781003401827-7

Strategic and Tactical Considerations

Crisis communication researchers and practitioners recommend that the form of communication during a crisis should be quick, consistent, and open (Coombs, 2019). Health crises like epidemics and pandemics require concerted efforts in crisis and emergency risk communication, primarily focusing on instructional information (Sturges, 1994). When there is a threat to public safety, people need urgent information about how they can protect themselves physically (Ndlela, 2019; Quarantelli, 1988). It is therefore important to be quick in crisis communications because viruses spread fast. In the age of digital communication, information spreads faster than ever before, thereby reducing the amount of time authorities have for planning and responding. Coombs (2019) posits that any discussions of crisis communication should include issues of *form, strategy*, and *content*. The form of communication pertains to the tactical aspect of communication and how the response should be presented. Effective communication is that which is quick and timely delivered to the intended audience. The speed of communication in a crisis is meant to avoid creating a void that can soon be filled by other competing messages. A silent response suggests that an organization is not in control and it allows others to take control of the situation (Coombs, 2019). Responding quickly is also a sign that those responsible for managing the crisis are prepared to respond to the emergency. Even when one does not have all the information at hand, communicating fast will indicate who has ownership of the crisis. Responding fast also creates long-lasting impressions on the audience. Some researchers argue that the first message received by the audience sets the stage for all future related messages (Covello, 2003). Another recommendation is that the messages should be consistent. Inconsistent messages will likely confuse the audience, create anxiety, and also diminish the risk experts' credibility. Consistency is essential to build up the credibility of the sources during a pandemic. Unfortunately, the pandemic exposed glaring inconsistences from the scientific community, resulting in some audience groups dismissing some health messages. The third recommendation is openness and honesty in communication. There are other characteristics that have been used to define what an effective message should possess such as clarity, appropriateness of tone, empathy, and relevance. This also includes messages that are free from technical jargon, that is, easy to understand.

The message should also have a focus on strategy and clearly indicate the desired outcomes (Coombs, 2019). What is the goal of risk communication? Is it to educate, advocate, or promote decision-making? In a pandemic, the initial objective is to minimize transmissions of the virus and hence minimize harm to individuals. The objective would also include efforts to promote psychological safety during the pandemic. Clear and frequent communication can reduce the uncertainty that often contributes to anxiety and the feeling of unsafety. The content of the messages focuses on what actually is said during a crisis (ibid.) The formulation of risk messages depends on the senders' intentions, be it instructing, educating, or persuasion.

Practice has shown that it is a daunting task to communicate messages quickly and maintain consistency due to the fluidity of the context. The COVID-19 pandemic has been unique in many ways. The spread of the virus has been gradual: very slow in the beginning or even non-existent in some areas. How then could authorities communicate quickly an invisible risk that was considered remote or non-existent? For most countries, there was no perceived immediate crisis or emergency, and hence less or delayed responses in some countries. The World Health Organization (WHO) noted the "alarming levels of inaction" by governments around the world (WHO, 2020: n.pag.). The inaction might have been caused by the fact that some countries had not registered a single case of infection. In Africa and Latin America, for example, the spread of information about the coronavirus superseded the virus itself. The pandemic generated a huge demand for information at a time when some countries had not yet recorded a single case of COVID-19 and local authorities did not have much risk information, if any, to give to the public, thus leading to an information crisis. The information crisis is manifested in various forms, such as the form and types of messages, the source of messages, the directions of message flow and the number of messages, information-seeking and -sharing behaviours, or the issues of truth and trust.

Information-Poor Context

One of the major challenges to risk and crisis communication during an unpredictable public health crisis is the deficiency of knowledge. During the onset of the coronavirus pandemic, very little was known or confirmed about the nature of the virus, its characteristics, and how it would evolve. This phenomenon is common in crises, aptly defined by Coombs (2019) as "information-poor and knowledge-poor situations" (p. 118). Public health authorities require huge amounts of information and scientifically proven facts about the new virus in order to create meaningful messages for the public. In situations like this, there is pressure for authorities to acquire information and process it into knowledge quickly and accurately in a seemingly unpredictable and rapidly changing environment. In the presence of a real threat to public health and the absence of any known medication or vaccine against the virus, communication is one of the pivotal measures for crisis containment. In other words, public health communication is central to addressing the pandemic. Yet, for some countries, the disease was on the shores and no one could predict its trajectory, where it would land, and what consequences it carried. When diseases are known, public health communicators can provide clear information about the disease and offer clear directives about how to avoid infection. This was not the case with the unpredictable coronavirus.

At the same time, when a public health emergency like an epidemic or a pandemic looms, people naturally seek information that will give them knowledge about the health risk they face and what actions they need to take to protect their lives. They turn to all possible sources of information – radio, newspapers, television, social media, family and friends – seeking information, knowledge, and answers to their numerous questions. First, the public wants to understand the virus itself. What is this virus? How is it transmitted? How does it spread? Who is at risk of contracting it? What are the symptoms? What are short- and long-term health impacts? Is there any cure for the disease? What is its mortality rate? Second, the public wants to know what they should do to protect themselves against the virus. What should they do to protect their health and life? What are the best ways to prevent contracting the virus? The questions might appear straightforward; however, public health authorities faced several challenges in providing timely and accurate risk messages to the public. This scenario creates an urgent need to fulfil the information needs of the public. Failure to do so creates an information vacuum, which will most likely be filled by others, some with half-truths and deceptive intentions.

Risk Information Vacuum

If risk information does not reach its intended recipients in time, a "risk information vacuum" can emerge. A risk information vacuum arises when "those who are conducting the evolving scientific research and assessments for high-profile risks make no special effort to communicate the results being obtained regularly and effectively to the public" (Powell & Leiss, 1997). Powell and Leiss (1997) postulate that a risk information vacuum is the result of that failure to implement good risk communication practices. Failures in risk communication lead to rumours and the spread of fear. In the era of fast communications, especially social media, such a risk communication vacuum can quickly be filled by other message sources. If the organization in charge is slow in communicating risks, other people can fill that gap and strengthen their position regarding the risk issues. As evidenced during the pandemic, the dearth of information from authoritative sources created a huge information vacuum that was soon filled by other voices and narratives of experiences on distant shores.

Effective risk communication can be utilized to fill this vacuum and translate the language of experts into something the public can more readily understand (Nielson, Kleffner, & Lee, 2005). Powell and Leiss (1997) define a good risk communication practice as communication that seeks to reconcile the language of expert risk assessment and public risk perception by, for example, translating the scientific findings and probabilistic risk assessment into understandable terms; explaining the uncertainty ranges, knowledge gaps; addressing the issue of building credibility and trust; understanding the public's perspectives on the risk issue; acknowledging that questions arising from the public are often quite different from those posed by the experts; and analysing the conditions needed for allowing the public to acquire needed information, skills, and participatory opportunities (Powell & Leiss, 1997, p. 30).

Success in risk communication is achieved when an organization has succeeded in communicating risk information to intended audiences, thereby earning their trust and most importantly, avoiding the development of a risk information vacuum. Effective risk communication also involves the ability of an organization to persuade segments of audiences. Powell and Leiss (1997) note that statements about risks by various parties are treated as "messages" intended to persuade others to believe or to do something.

Message Purpose: What Messages Hope to Achieve

An important consideration in risk and crisis communication during the pandemic is the alignment of the messages to the overall strategic objectives. Strategy relates to the overall crisis management goals. Goals indicate the most preferred outcome of communication or what the communicator seeks to achieve. Objectives reflect the desired outcomes, and these are guided by the strategy. Objectives add specific details as to how the overall goals can be achieved and they do so by defining specific targets to accomplish the strategic goals (Sutherland, 2021). Ideally, these objectives should follow the key specific, measurable, achievable, realistic, and time-specific (SMART) criteria (Freberg, 2019). Communication strategies fall within two broad categories: short- and long-term strategies (or ongoing strategies). Short-term strategies are developed to guide communication activities around a specific event, while ongoing strategies can be longer, depending on the trajectory of the pandemic.

Risk and crisis management messages are generally intended to support overall national crisis management strategies. The pandemic required crisis management measures across the world. However, as noted in the above chapters, different countries and regions adopted different pandemic strategies, from zero COVID-19 strategies in countries like China and herd immunity in Sweden to more relaxed approaches in some African and Latin American countries. Some countries later adjusted their original strategies. The different pandemic strategies not only led to different outcomes, but also influenced the messages used to support the chosen national strategies. It is not surprising that the global coronavirus pandemic messages were characterized by contradictory messages.

Message Presentation Formats

Many messages were generated during the COVID-19 pandemic, unlike in any other public health crisis before. With a plethora of communication channels to use in the communication of the pandemic, different presentation formats were used in the rhetorical construction of the COVID-19 pandemic risk. Risk is about probabilities, and communication of probability estimates influences people's stance toward risk. Uncertainty is one of the defining characteristics of probabilities (i.e. the likelihood of an event happening). Lipkus (2007) argues that the probability dimension is perhaps the most difficult dimension of risk to convey and understand. Visschers et al. (2009) also note that communicating probability information about risks to the public is more difficult than expected. Similarly, Ancker et al. (2006) note that one of the many challenges to risk communication with the public is the difficulty in expressing quantitative information in an easily comprehensible form. Waters et al. (2006) argue that the way in which messages are formatted influences the degree to which laypeople can understand them. It is therefore essential to use aids and brief summaries in order to improve understanding of messages. Using a combination of formats can improve the effectiveness of messages.

Risk and crisis communication messages during the COVID-19 pandemic were presented in various formats – numerical, verbal descriptions and visualization of frequencies, percentages, base rates and proportions, and cumulative probabilities. Verbal probability information, numerical, graphs, and risk ladders aided the message strategies of the public health authorities. Table 7.1 shows a cursory overview of some message presentation formats.

Table 7.1 Message presentation formats

Numerical	Verbal	Visualized models
Range of percentage	**Use of descriptive terms**	**Use of graphs, diagrams**
<1%	Extremely unlikely	Infographics
1–10%	Very unlikely	Pie charts
10–33 %	Unlikely	Graphs
33–66 %	Medium likelihood	Bar diagrams
66–90 %	Likely	Cartography
90–99 %	Very likely	Pictograms
>99 %	Virtually certain	Cartoons
Use of plain numbers	Almost certain	
10	Possible	
50	Rare	
	Extremely unlikely	
	Almost never	
	Seldom	
	Infrequent	
	Sometimes	
	Even chance	
	More often than not	
	Often	

Numerical Communication: The Power and Politics of Numbers

Numerical communication involves the use of numbers in communication. The public can be informed that they have a certain percentage chance of getting COVID-19 after exposure to the virus or 5 in 100 chance of getting the virus. Lipkus (2007, p. 699) notes that numbers have several appealing qualities. First, numbers are precise and as such, lead to more accurate perceptions of risk than the use of probability phrases and graphical displays. Second, numbers convey an aura of scientific credibility. Third, numbers can be converted from one metric to another (e.g. 10 % = 1 out of 10). Fourth, numbers can be verified for accuracy, and finally, numbers can be computed using an algorithm to provide a summary score.

While numerical formats might have these advantages over other formats, they appeal to a highly literate public. Readers with limited numeracy skills would find it difficult to make sense of numerical information. Patt and Dessai (2005) note how communicating probabilities is beset with challenges of interpretation. Actors understand and interpret probabilistic information differently and people choose to ignore probabilistic information that is too complicated for them. Numbers may not be enough to convey intended meanings. As Lipkus (2007) aptly notes, a single number may not be enough to convey the magnitude of risk. The same number does not have the same meaning across different contexts. Universal cognitive limitations cause biases in interpreting numerical probabilities (Ancker et al., 2006).

The COVID-19 risk communications have highlighted the significance of numbers and stats in the rhetorical constructions of the crisis narratives. COVID-19 data provided a springboard for widely diverse agendas, be it the support of pandemic management strategic goals and tactics, economic interests, or political scores. Authorities relied on numbers to make important decisions like shutdowns or reopening of society, travel restrictions, and so forth. Governments used numbers to construct their stories and persuade people to take certain actions. The pandemic management has been, to a large extent, data-driven. An entry in Magnifirm (2020) argues that COVID-19 can be regarded as one of the biggest data stories of the century. It notes that "many countries locked down their citizens with zero or handfuls of initial cases in hospitals, in what can be seen as a triumph of math and science over natural social gregariousness and economic interest". Flatten-the-curve (FTC) persuasive narratives were built around numbers and mathematical models. FTC refers to the strategy adopted in the early phases of the pandemic to slow down and spread out the outbreak dynamic. Mat Daud (2022) posits that FTC was a succinct way of communicating an important public health message that physical distancing and other public health measures would reduce the peak number of cases. The overall goal of the FTC was to prevent the healthcare system from being overwhelmed.

Like data, COVID-19 numbers could be used to promote different agendas. The political aspects of numbers centre on the way the numbers are collected and analysed and their intended use. Their use in decision-making and comparison of leadership effectiveness makes them a potential source of political contest. Numerical information has been a source of contention during the COVID-19 pandemic. In addition to the general problem of presentation format, numerical communication of risk has been saddled with issues of accuracy, relevance, and effectiveness. Governments around the world responded differently on how the data about the disease was collected, collated, and shared with the country's citizens and the global stakeholders. Countries adopted different testing policies and registering of infections and death, hence different outcomes.

The selectiveness of what to share and not share concerning confirmed cases and deaths led to controversies around statistical information and its presentation. The accuracy of the figures was questioned by governments and citizens alike. The number of infections and deaths reflected negatively on the political leadership of the crisis, hence the lack of transparency on data that reflected negatively on the ruling authorities. Some leaders manipulated or downplayed the numbers to build or suit certain narratives or downplay criticism. In the US, the data on COVID-19 was a centre of contention with the trading of accusations of undercounting, manipulation, exaggeration, and bias, reflective of the political polarization in the country. In an interview with Associated Press, then-President Donald Trump argued that the US had better coronavirus death numbers than other countries if counted as a percentage of cases, not the total population.[1] Big powers like China have also been accused of not being transparent with the numbers. The accuracy of the Chinese data has been questioned. In the wake of a surge in COVID-19 cases towards the end of 2022, there were concerns that China was hiding its COVID-19 infection death toll following its adoption of a narrower criterion for identifying deaths caused by COVID-19.

In Sub-Saharan countries, reliable data is difficult to collect, given the limited resources for reliable economic and census data in general (Mansell, Lee Rhea, & Murray, 2023). Authoritarian governments generally avoid transparency. In their research on Nigeria, Ernest-Samuel and Uduma (2022) note general controversies regarding the number of infections and mistrust between the Nigerian Centre for Disease Control (NCDC) and state governments. They note how the squabbles around the accuracy of the figures engendered doubts and a loss of public trust. In Zimbabwe, the audiences complained that the government was just dumping statistics without giving them information on what the public could do to protect themselves (Kembo & Bothma, 2023). The statistics were not entirely relevant to the audience whose priority was seeking information and knowledge on what to do in order to protect themselves from the virus. A potential weakness of numeric information used alone is that it lacks completeness and explanations, as noted in the case of Zimbabwe. People's level of numeracy has a bearing on the effectiveness of numerical information.

While there are some advantages in numerical communication of risk, the presentation format should be tailored to the audiences, their numeracy, and their ability to interpret probability information. There are various issues to consider when communicating numerical risks to ordinary audiences. Numbers should easily be understood by the intended audience. Correct numerical information in a complex numerical format will undoubtedly not yield the intended response. Numerical presentation formats should ideally be dependent on the context (Siegrist, 1997) and should be accompanied by "adjunct aids" such as highlighting and summaries (Fischhoff, Bostrom, & Quadrel, 1993). Poorly presented information can have a negative effect on required responses. Statistic information alone is insufficient for communicating risk to the public during a pandemic.

To increase the understandability and efficacy of numerical messages, researchers (Lipkus, 2007; Waters et al., 2006) offer a set of recommendations on the presentation format:

- Simplify the calculations
- Be consistent in the use of numeric formats
- Use of the same numeric denominators
- Use round numbers and avoid the use of decimals
- Numbers close to zero will at times be dismissed as representing no risk (e.g. 1% or less)

Verbal Communication of Risk

Verbal communication of risks relies on the use of linguistic terms to describe the risk. Terms such as *extremely unlikely, very unlikely, unlikely*, and many others can be used to describe the degree of risk. Researchers have assessed the efficiency of verbal terms in the communication of risk and probabilities. The advantage of using text to denote the risk is that they are easy and natural to use and can convey the level, source, and imprecision of uncertainty (Erev & Cohen, 1990; Lipkus, 2007). In their survey on the preferences and reasons for communicating probabilistic information in verbal or numerical terms, Wallsten et al. (1993) found that respondents who endorsed verbal information said that it was much easier to use and understand, more natural and personal, and reflect the degree of precision in the communicator's opinion.

However, one of the major weaknesses of using phrases is that there is currently no standardized format and phrases are open to various meanings. Differences between linguistics formulations can be perceived differently. Olchowska-Kotala (2019) has noted the challenges inherent in communicating messages to patients. Formulations such as "this is a bad message" versus "this message is not good" or "this is a good message" versus "this message is not bad" and "risk is high" versus "the risk is not low" can convey different meanings and significantly affect how the receiver perceives the risk. Context and the individual attributes of the receiver influence the interpretation. Individual differences in the use and interpretation of these terms are large. Hence, if the goal of communication is to achieve precision in risk estimates, then the higher degree of variability of interpretation will negatively affect that (Lipkus, 2007). Challenges also arise through the translation as the terms might not have the same meaning in local languages.

Visual Presentation

The COVID-19 pandemic communication was hugely supported by all sorts of visualized information, both static and interactive visualization. Visual formats like graphics provide another format for presenting risk communication. Graphical presentations include several displays such as bar graphs, pie charts, histograms, ovals, risk ladders, dots, films, cartoons, and so forth. Visualising information has become a prominent mode for making information "meaning-ful" and discovering important relationships within data sets (Salvo, 2012). Jones (2015) postulates that visuals have become a required adjunct to many complex arguments. The advantages of graphical displays are that they make it easier to visualize trends, variations, and comparisons. Graphical material makes it easier to summarize a great deal of data and reveal patterns in these data that would otherwise go undetected (Cleveland & McGill, 1984). Visual material also attracts the readers' attention because they are visually interesting and exploit rapid, automatic visual perception skills (Cleveland & McGill, 1985). Theories on perception hold that translating numeric information into visual formats allows that information to be "filtered and evaluated" intuitively by readers, who can then make perceptual comparisons such as size and orientation (Brasseur, 2003; Jones, 2015). People also tend to perceive data visualizations about COVID-19 as objective representations of their numbers because they associate charts with logical arguments and scientific enlightenment (Cairo, 2019). Other researchers have noted the rhetorical potency imbued in information visualization (Rath, 2022).

However, Ancker et al. (2006) caution that communicators should not assume that all graphics are more intuitive than texts, as some aspects of graph interpretation also require effortful cognitive skills. Furthermore, the public frequently interprets graphs in ways that are not intended by their designers (ibid.). Just like any communication form, graphical displays have to be decoded by the audience. Lipkus (2007) notes that some of the disadvantages of graphical material or other displays are that data patterns may discourage people from attending to details like numbers, and poorly designed or complex graphical material may not be understandable by the general public. In their research on health marketing in Zimbabwe during COVID-19, Kembo and Bothma (2023) note how the Ministry of Health's poor graphic presentation irked some members of the audience. The daily situational report disseminated by the ministry in the digital media was an unclear, black-and-white document that was not readable most of the time. The graphical material disseminated by the ministry was not designed with digital media in mind, but they were merely scanned in a low-resolution scanning equipment, resulting in the blurring of text.

Since the COVID-19 pandemic was declared, digital communication media has been awash with graphical displays of complex statistics about the pandemic. While the graphs have been helping in visualising the trajectory of the virus, they are prone to manipulation. Glen (2020) notes that while graphs are a great tool to appeal to a wide audience, they are often used to deliberately mislead and not to inform, as evidenced by their creative use to distort COVID-19 facts. Media outlets, pushing for certain narratives or lack of appropriate science journalism skills produced misleading arguments around COVID-19.

In her article "Misrepresenting COVID-19: Lying With Charts During the Second Golden Age of Data Design", Doan (2020) examines various forms of data visualizations about COVID-19 and highlights three ways in which charts can mislead the viewers: (a) displaying inadequate data, (b) manipulating scales and visual distance, and (c) omitting contextual labels. Some of the graphical material was visually manipulated to mislead the public and push for other agendas. Kotsehub (2020) posits that the Argentinian, Russian, and the Georgian (US State) media manipulated the graphs either because of incompetence in statistics or intentionally to paint a better picture of their country. Kotsehub (2020) shows how the visualization of statistics in graphs can paint an entirely different picture due to the manipulation of bar sizes and improper use of scaling. Glancing at the visual (bars) without looking at the numerical values creates a wrong impression to the reader. In the case of the US State of Georgia, the public was quick to spot the manipulation and voiced their concern, resulting in the withdrawal of the graph and an apology by the governor's spokesperson. Apparently, the graphs were presented not only to inform but also to fit a particular narrative.

It is therefore vital for the audience to take a critical stance at the information presented in the graphs to ascertain if the visuals match the numerics. It should however be noted that fact-checking charts and visual presentation is not an easy task and require a certain level of numeracy. An individual who lacks appropriate skills will be misled by visual information. In his book *How Charts Lie: Getting Smarter about Visual Information* (2019), Cairo explores the negative – and the positive – influences that charts have on the public's perception of truth. He argues that charts, infographics, and diagrams can also deceive intentionally or unintentionally. In a digital environment where everyone with an online presence is a publisher, inaccurate or misleading visualization spread faster and wider and informs public conversation, which is increasingly driven by numbers (ibid.). Cairo emphasizes that to be informed, citizens must be able to decode and use visual information.

The three formats of presentation presented above have both positive and negative aspects. Audiences' preferences and skills have a bearing on the effectiveness of the message. If the audience lack basic numerical skills, they cannot properly interpret the information presented to them. To alleviate the challenges associated with the presenting formats, verbal descriptions can be combined with numerical data or visualization. People need help in interpreting not only what the numbers are but also what they actually mean (Olchowska-Kotala, 2019). Visuals do not explain themselves (Lindgren, 2021). The risk message should be tailored to the intended audiences, taking into consideration their linguistic skills. The readability of the risk messages should match the target audience's comprehension levels. The choice of message delivery modes should be informed by the target audience's communication habits.

Why Context Matters

The choice of presentation format should be guided by the context, that is, the environment and situation where communication takes place. Visschers et al. (2009) argue that the effect of these presentation formats depends not only on the type of format but also on the context in which the format is used. Visschers et al. (2009) argue that risk communication practitioners should not only concentrate on the presentation format of the probability information but also on the situation in which this message is communicated. The context of communication has a bearing on the comprehension of the message. Context influences not only the reception of the message but also its meaning. Context also determines the communication alternatives. Communicators should take into consideration the rhetorical situations of their intended audiences.

Conclusion

The creation of messages during a pandemic should be informed and guided by strategic and tactical considerations. Messages seek to fulfil several tasks during a pandemic, be it to inform the public, educate or persuade individuals to adopt risk-averting behaviours or comply with recommendations. Considerations should be given to message presentation formats based on the complexity of the information presented and the audience's attributes such as their literacy levels. Messages should ideally be tailored to the audience and the context of communication.

Note

1 https://www.youtube.com/watch?v=NmrEfQG6pIg (Accessed 02.03.2023).

References

Ancker, J. S., Senathirajah, Y., Kukafka, R., & Starren, J. B. (2006). Design features of graphs in health risk communication: A systematic review. *Journal of the American Medical Informatics Association, 13*(6), 608–618. doi:10.1197/jamia.M2115

Brasseur, L. E. (2003). *Visualizing Technical Information: A Cultural Critique*. Amityville, NY: Baywood.

Cairo, A. (2019). *How Charts Lie: Getting Smarter about Visual Information*. New York: W.W. Norton.

Cleveland, W. S., & McGill, R. (1984). Graphical perception: Theory, Experimentation, and application to the development of graphical methods. *Journal of the American Statistical Association, 79*(387), 531–554. doi:10.2307/2288400

Cleveland, W. S., & McGill, R. (1985). Graphical perception and graphical methods for analyzing scientific data. *Science, 229*(4716), 828–833. doi:10.1126/science.229.4716.828

Coombs, W. T. (2019). *Ongoing Crisis Communication: Planning, Managing, and Responding* (5 ed.). Los Angeles, CA: Sage.

Covello, V. T. (2003). Best Practices in public health risk and crisis communication. *Journal of Health Communication, 8*(suppl), 5–8. doi:10.1080/713851971

Doan, S. (2020). Misrepresenting COVID-19: Lying with charts during the second golden age of data design. *Journal of Business and Technical Communication, 35*(1), 73–79. doi:10.1177/1050651920958392

Erev, I., & Cohen, B. L. (1990). Verbal versus numerical probabilities: Efficiency, biases, and the preference paradox. *Organizational Behavior Human Decision Processes, 45*(1), 1–18. doi:10.1016/0749-5978(90)90002-Q

Ernest-Samuel, G. C., & Uduma, N. E. (2022). Nigerian government and management of news and information on the coronavirus pandemic. *14*(Media and the Coronavirus Pandemic in Africa (Part Three)), 143–158. doi:10.1386/jams_00070_1

Fischhoff, B., Bostrom, A., & Quadrel, M. J. (1993). Risk perception and communication. *Annual Review of Public Health, 14*(1), 183–203. doi:10.1146/annurev.pu.14.050193.001151

Freberg, K. (2019). *Social Media for Strategic Communication*. Los Angeles, CA: Sage.

Glen, S. (2020). The worst Covid-19 misleading graphs. Retrieved from https://www.datasciencecentral.com/the-worst-covid-19-misleading-graphs/

Jones, J. (2015). Information graphics and intuition: Heuristics as a techne for visualization. *Journal of Business and Technical Communication, 29*(3), 284–313. doi:10.1177/1050651915573943

Kembo, S., & Bothma, C. (2023). A critical review of health marketing in Zimbabwe during COVID-19. *Journal of African Media Studies, 15*(1), 91–109.

Kotsehub, N. (2020). Stopping COVID-19 with misleading graphs. Retrieved from https://towardsdatascience.com/stopping-covid-19-with-misleading-graphs-6812a61a57c9

Lindgren, C. A. (2021). Facts upon delivery: What is rhetorical about visualized models?, *35*(1), 65–72. doi:10.1177/1050651920958499

Lipkus, I. M. (2007). Numeric, verbal, and visual formats of conveying health risks: Suggested best practices and future recommendations. *Medical Decision Making: An International Journal of the Society for Medical Decision Making, 27*(5), 696–713. doi:10.1177/0272989x07307271

Magnifirm. (2020). Justifying a shutdown: Covid-19 and the data story of the century. Retrieved from https://www.magnifirm.com/articles/data-stories/marketing-coronavirus-lockdown-to-the-public-the-covid19-data-backstory/

Mansell, J., Lee Rhea, C., & Murray, G. R. (2023). Predicting the issuance of COVID-19 stay-at-home orders in Africa: Using machine learning to develop insight for health policy research. *International Journal of Disaster Risk Reduction*, 103598. doi:10.1016/j.ijdrr.2023.103598

Mat Daud, A. A. (2022). Five common misconceptions regarding flattening-the-curve of COVID-19. *History and Philosophy of the Life Sciences, 44*(3), 41. doi:10.1007/s40656-022-00522-x

Morgan, M. G., & Lave, L. (1990). Ethical considerations in risk communication. *Risk Analysis, 10*, 355–358.

Ndlela, M. (2019). *Crisis Communication. A Stakeholder Perspective*. Cham: Switzerland: Palgrave Macmillan.

Nielson, N. L., Kleffner, A. E., & Lee, R. B. (2005). The evolution of the role of risk communication in effective risk management. *Risk Management and Insurance Review, 8*(2), 279–289.

Olchowska-Kotala, A. (2019). Verbal descriptions accompanying numeric information about the risk: The valence of message and linguistic polarity. *Journal of Psycholinguistic Research, 48*(6), 1429–1439. doi:10.1007/s10936-019-09666-7

Patt, A., & Dessai, S. (2005). Communicating uncertainty: Lessons learned and suggestions for climate change assessment. *C. R. Geophysics, 337*, 425–441.

Powell, D. A., & Leiss, W. (1997). *Mad Cows and Mother's Milk: The Perils of Poor Risk Communication*. Montreal, QC: McGill-Queen's University Press.

Quarantelli, E. L. (1988). Disaster crisis management: A summary of research findings. *Journal of Management Studies, 32*(2), 24–29.

Rath, K. (2022). The rhetoric of Covid-19: Numbers and stats and maps – Oh My! *Communicatio, 48*(1), 1–27. doi:10.1080/02500167.2022.2058041

Salvo, M. J. (2012). Visual rhetoric and big data: Design of future communication. *Communication Design Quarterly, 1*(1), 37–40. doi:10.1145/2448917.2448925

Siegrist, M. (1997). Communicating low risk magnitudes: Incidence rates expressed as frequency versus rates expressed as probability. *Risk Analysis, 17*(4), 507–510. doi:10.1111/j.1539-6924.1997.tb00891.x

Sturges, D. L. (1994). Communicating through Crisis. *Management Communication Quarterly, 7*(3), 297–316. doi:10.1177/0893318994007003004

Sutherland, K. E. (2021). *Strategic Social Media Management: Theory and Practice*. Singapore: Palgrave Macmillan.

Visschers, V. H. M., Meertens, R. M., Passchier, W. W. F., & De Vries, N. N. K. (2009). Probability information in risk communication: A review of the research literature. *Risk Analysis, 29*(2), 267–287. doi:10.1111/j.1539-6924.2008.01137.x

Wallsten, T. S., Budescu, D. V., Zwick, R., & Kemp, S. M. (1993). Preferences and reasons for communicating probabilistic information in verbal or numerical terms. *Bulletin of the Psychonomic Society, 31*(2), 135–138. doi:10.3758/BF03334162

Waters, E. A., Weinstein, N. D., Colditz, G. A., & Emmons, K. (2006). Formats for improving risk communication in medical tradeoff decisions. *Journal of Health Communication, 11*(2), 167–182. doi:10.1080/10810730500526695

8   Audiences and Messages

Introduction

The coronavirus pandemic created an unprecedented need for governments to communicate with their citizens about the public health scare, actions taken to prevent and mitigate its impact, and what citizens should do to protect themselves and society in general. The pandemic carried both societal and individual risks and these had to be communicated to fearful audiences. Both the levels of societal risk (i.e. the estimates of total harm to the population in terms of the number of people getting infected and the numbers of fatalities) and individual risk (specific individuals exposed to the risk of harm or death) had to be taken into account in the risk and crisis communication messages. Governments had to justify their risk (in-)tolerability criteria and their risk reduction measures.

To prevent the spread of the virus, many governments adopted a range of measures such as restrictions on movement, social distancing, quarantine, isolation, and closure of non-essential institutions and services such as churches, schools, colleges, universities, and the travel and hospitality industries. These overarching measures had widespread implications across all strata of society and inevitably led to difficult debates (e.g. at political, cultural, or economic levels), disagreements, and sometimes disobedience. As such, the pandemic became a source of other spin-off crises. Alongside the health crisis, there emerged "economic crisis", "political crisis", "cultural crisis", and "moral crisis" (Fuchs, 2021). One can also add "humanitarian crisis" to this list of crises. Undoubtedly, the pandemic crisis led to another crisis that informs the bulk of this book, that is, the "information crisis".

This chapter focuses on the audiences of risk and crisis communication during the pandemic and the barriers to achieving the purposes of communication. The pandemic created an unprecedented need for governments to communicate with their citizens about the public health scare, actions taken to prevent and mitigate its impact, and what citizens should do to protect themselves and society in general. Yet, audiences today have become more diverse, fragmented, and multifaceted. Communicators today need to communicate to hugely varied and complex

DOI: 10.4324/9781003401827-8

audiences, including populations that are "hard-to-reach" and "hardly-reached". This chapter underlines the importance of understanding the rhetorical context, shaping how audiences interact and respond to messages.

The Audience

The audience is paramount in any communication process, and hence, understanding the audience for which the message is intended is crucial if risk communication is to succeed. In a crisis, communicators need to know their audiences so that they can best adapt and tailor the messages to target groups. Audience characteristics and context will have a bearing on the reception of messages. The audience of a risk message is not monolithic, but is diverse and complex. Communicators need to know whom the message is intended for before they can customize it to suit the audience's needs. Marketers are known for being savvy when it comes to finding the target audience for their products and services. They devote a great deal of their time segmenting and analysing their potential audiences – their preferences, behaviours, and attributes – before deciding who their real target audience are. They define a target group as a specific group of consumers most likely to buy their products and services. A target audience is imperative for any successful risk communication. As Freimuth et al. (2000) note, "the clearer the understanding of the audience for which the message is intended, the better the chance of developing an effective message" (p. 338). The goal of risk and crisis communication is after all to ensure that the target audience (1) hears the message; (2) understands its content; (3) internalizes or believes the salience of the message; (4) confirms their interpretation with others; and (5) act or respond to the message to save their life and property (Blanchard-Boehm, 1998). Yet the audiences in a pandemic are extremely diverse. They include individuals and groups with different backgrounds – educational, cultural, linguistic, religious, and many other differentiating factors such as age, income, place of residence, and profession. Any risk message will resonate differently with the audiences. Some groups might get the message but not understand it. Some might not even access the message due to inaccessible language or communication channels. Some might get the message but are distrustful of the source. Some will get the message and put their own meaning into it. Some will perceive these messages as not relevant. Some groups are likely to be overseen, less prioritized, or simply ignored. Some messages might not even reach all the groups intended by the communicator.

Multivocality and Multiple Publics

A crisis of this magnitude attracts the multiple "voices" seeking to communicate in various ways – "some voices communicate *to* each other, other voices communicate *with* each other, some voices communicate *against* each other, or *past* each other, and finally they are voices that just communicate *about* each other" (Frandsen & Johansen, 2017, p. 149). Public authorities seeking to convey their messages to the public had to contend with the competition of multiple voices in the digital public sphere. In addition, public authorities are confronted with inherent challenges of making sense of the threat and co-ordinating their communication messages. The realities of a global pandemic are such that public authorities within countries and around the world differ in their understanding of the risk, approaches, and strategies for crisis management; hence the resultant polarization in their core messages. Competing and conflicting messages inevitably reach the audiences. The media institutions, which often have a mammoth task of disseminating information to the public during a crisis, are undergoing unprecedented changes due to changes in digital communication. The media no longer have the monopoly to filter messages intended for the public. In social media, unfiltered messages flourish, making it even more difficult for people to know what is relevant and correct.

Health crises have multiple stakeholders and hence voices. Health risks and crises represent highly complex stakeholder dynamics occupying different levels within the national and international health chain system. Stakeholders in a health crisis play different roles about others and each has a different viewpoint on the care system, hence different information needs. These stakeholders include *policymakers*, that is, those who establish the framework with which health services are delivered. This can be ministries of health, agencies, or any other jurisdictional entity with responsibility for health prevention and care within and across national boundaries. The other key stakeholders are *service providers*, that is, those who operationalize preventive care and care delivery services. Stakeholders such as *industry providers* include producers (e.g. medical supplies and pharmaceuticals), purchasers, and providers. The other group of stakeholders consists of the *general public* and the *patients*. All stakeholders involved in the reduction of risk, for example, organizations charged with public health, need to find a way to communicate with their stakeholders about current and developing risks.

The Rhetorical Situation

Political leadership and public health authorities across the world had to contend with the challenges of persuading their citizens to adopt risk-mitigating behaviours. The authorities' communication abilities, personalities, and leadership styles were pivotal in the pandemic management, all within a context of extraordinary complexity and uncertainty. Aristotle's rhetorical triangle provides a good analytic tool for understanding the complexity of the risk and crisis communication context during the pandemic. The three central elements that inform persuasive communication in Aristotle's rhetorical triangle are *ethos* (appeal to credibility and ethics), *pathos* (appeal to emotions and feelings), and *logos*

AUDIENCE

PURPOSE

SPEAKER   Context   MESSAGE

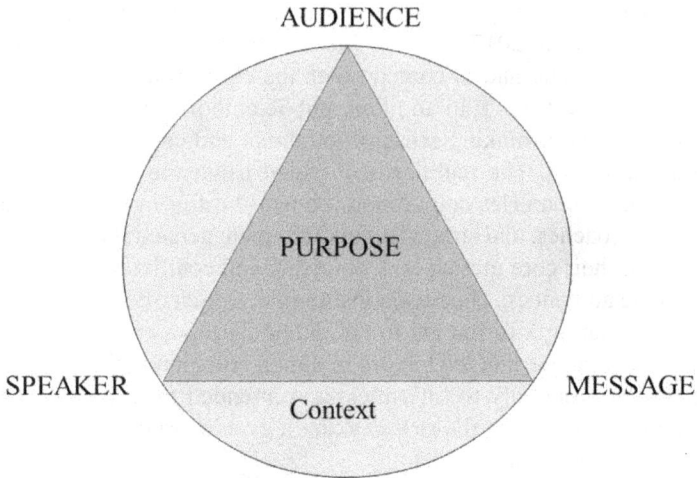

Figure 8.1 The rhetorical situation.

(appeal to logic and reason). Messages of persuasion can be based on the appeal to emotions or rational appeals to logic by using statistics, figures, and real stories. The communicator draws on rhetorical tools to attract attention while conveying the messages. Communication takes place within a rhetorical situation that is composed of several primary elements: (1) the communicator and his motivations; (2) the audience; (3) the purpose of the text; (4) the message; and (5) the context in which communication takes places. Figure 8.1 illustrates the relationship between these components.

The Cultural Context

The rhetorical context describes the setting and circumstances surrounding the pandemic risk and crisis communication. The risk communication process did not take place in a vacuum. It was shaped by all that exists around them – the audiences, their language, culture, and the social-political and economic configurations. There are various forms of denoting context. The concept can be used to describe the physical setting of communication (physical location and time), the temporal context (that refers to past experiences and expectations), and the socio-physical context (that relates to the people's emotional states and relationships). All these factors have played an important role in shaping the audiences, their message reception, and compliance or non-compliance. This section focuses mainly on the cultural aspects of the rhetorical context.

Culture provides an overall framework for understanding the society in which human communication takes place. It encompasses thought systems, emotions, and norms of behaviour. Culture includes aspects of language, social norms, beliefs, technology, economics, politics, educational systems, and so forth. Culture is hence an important puzzle in risk and communication during a pandemic. In a nutshell, culture affects how people communicate. Previous studies on culture highlight some of the national cultural traits that possibly inform the audience's reaction to pandemic messages (Cialdini & Goldstein, 2004; Huynh, 2020; Triandis, 1989). Triandis (1989) used the notion of cultural complexity to refer to the many attributes of some cultures. In their study, Gelfand et al. (2011) differentiate between cultures that are tight (these cultures have strong norms and a low tolerance for deviant behaviour) and cultures that are loose (these cultures have weak social norms and a high tolerance for deviant behaviour). Social norms, that is, implicit or explicit social rules that guide individual behaviours, are a glue that keeps society together and in many ways determine the success of communication interventions. In their research on the relationship between cultural tightness-looseness and COVID-19 cases and deaths, Gelfand et al. (2021) conclude that tight groups co-operate much faster under threat and have higher survival rates than loose groups. They argue that nations that are tight and abide by strict norms have had more success than those that are looser (ibid.). Their citizens are more likely to willingly co-operate under threat. For example, in Taiwan, "increased self-regulation and voluntary norm abidance with physical distancing, wearing masks, and avoiding large crowds enabled the country to keep both the infection and mortality rates low without shutting down the economy entirely" (Gelfand et al., 2021, p. 142). Cultural variations explain why certain countries were more successful than others in the face of a similar pandemic threat. Understanding the cultural tightness-looseness of a country can help guide interventions aimed at addressing future collective threats (ibid.)

Hofstede's cultural diversity model provides insights into how we can understand culture (Hofstede, 2001). Hofstede's three widely used dimensions are individualism versus collectivism, power distance, and uncertainty avoidance. The individual versus collectivism relates to the degree to which the community reinforces individual or collective goals. Individualistic cultures give priority to personal goals over the goals of the collective, while collectivist cultures make no distinctions between personal and collective goals (Triandis, 1989). Dimension of power distance denotes the difference between those with power and those without. It also relates to how people are willing to accept a difference of power. Collectivist cultures tend to be high in power distance (Triandis, 1989). Uncertainty avoidance captures the cultural perception of the uncertain, unknown, and unstructured situations (Hofstede, 2001). Different cultures react and behave differently to threat perception. These cultural dimensions and distinctions are useful in understanding communication because they influence the audience's perception of risk and risk messages. The cultural context has an enormous bearing on the decoding of messages to such an extent that a communicator who does not understand the context is bound to fail.

The pandemic taught us that messages and recommendations do not have the same meaning across cultures. One of the key recommendations during the pandemic was social distancing. It was scientifically envisaged that "individual behaviour would be crucial to control the spread of COVID-19" (Anderson, Heesterbeek, Klinkenberg, & Hollingsworth, 2020) and keeping a distance from others was recommended. The implication of these on social distancing, as Huynh (2020) points out, is that while Asian countries have applied strict and punishable rules on social distancing, European countries were likely to recommend people to stay at home, given that loose cultures prioritize privacy as well as the freedom of each individualism. Comparing Asian, European, Latin American, Oceania, and Australian on the observation of social distancing, Huynh (2020) shows that people coming from countries with "risk-adverse" tend to stay more at home. The study shows that cultural factors can influence the efficiency of social distancing. Cultural differences matter for social distancing during a pandemic, as people might have different perceptions and viewpoints with regards to COVID-19. Social norms heterogeneously influence human behaviours on social distancing.

Cultural context plays a pivotal role in human behaviours, compliance, and conformity (Cialdini & Goldstein, 2004). In their research on culture and COVID-19, Nair et al. (2022) infer that:

> The cultural dimension of collectivism is positively related to higher engagement in COVID-19 protective behaviours such as mask wearing and social contact avoidance, compared to more individualistic cultures.
>
> (p. 1213)

In collectivist countries such as China, South Korea, and Singapore, there appeared to have been more adherence to lockdown rules (Chen, Frey, & Presidente, 2021) compared to individualistic Western Europe and North America. Individualistic contexts had to weigh up COVID-19 restrictions with personal freedoms and autonomy. It should be noted that within the US, there are huge cultural variations between states.

On the dimension of power distance, Nair et al. (2022) conclude that:

> Adherence to health policy guidelines and government mandates and restrictions to curb the spread of COVID-19 is higher in high power distance countries than in low power distance countries.
>
> (p. 1215)

Nair et al. (2022) argue that the differences in behavioural responses in terms of audience abiding by preventive measures during the pandemic can be attributed to power distance norms prevailing in the country. They conclude that contexts with higher power distance have an advantage in containing the pandemic compared to those with lower power distance. Gupta et al. (2022) argue that individuals in higher power distance contexts are willing to acknowledge the role of government and willingly comply with many tough measures such as protracted lockdowns. On the cultural dimension of uncertainty avoidance, Nair et al. (2022) conclude that:

> Cultures low in uncertainty avoidance are more likely to have a tolerance for varied risk mitigation strategies requiring behavioral changes than cultures high in uncertainty avoidance.
>
> (p. 1216)

The uncertainty avoidance dimension of a national culture has implications for COVID-19 mitigating behaviours. Nair et al. cite the case of Germany, a high uncertainty avoidance society, which witnessed several anti-lockdown protests during the pandemic.

Several empirical studies highlight the significance of context, in particular the cultural dimensions of a country in the mitigation of the spread of the pandemic. A country's national culture shapes the behaviours of the audiences; hence the communication context for risk and crisis communication. National cultures, power distance, individualism/collectivism, and other cultural traits shape people's behaviours. Cultural factors undoubtedly explain the variations in the successes and failures of COVID-19 containment measures. Communicators should hence be attentive to the contexts in which their messages are communicated. The cultural aspects of the rhetorical context undoubtedly inform risk and crisis communication audiences.

Hard-to-Reach Audience

In any crisis, public authorities endeavour to reach everyone with the information that they need to be aware of the lurking dangers and to make informed decisions. For various reasons, as evidenced during past crises, some audiences are more difficult to reach than others. The consequences of failing to reach everyone can be catastrophic. The hurricane which hit the Gulf Coast of the USA in August 2005, resulting in more than 1800 deaths, became one of the deadliest hurricanes in the history of the USA. The communication failures experienced during the disaster illustrate the challenges of communicating with hard-to-reach audiences. As Froonjian and Garnett (2013) aptly put it:

> The importance of communicating with the hard-to-reach in times of emergencies and natural disasters could not be illustrated more powerfully than by the devastation wreaked by Hurricane Katrina in late August 2005.
>
> (p. 831)

Hurricane Katrina was as much a communication disaster as it was a natural disaster. Communication was compromised at all levels, including communication with the so-called hard-to-reach audiences. Communication barriers in reaching vulnerable and isolated populations, especially African Americans and other ethnic minorities, is one of the factors that accounted for the high number of casualties. Many African Americans failed to evacuate due to communication failures and lack of trust in the authorities.

African Americans are referred to in several literatures as hard-to-reach audiences. Who are hard-to-reach audiences? The term hard-to-reach is commonly used to describe "individuals or groups whom an institution finds difficult to contact or engage for a particular purpose" (Brackertz, Zwart, Meredyth, & Ralston, 2005). In the field of health communication, the label "hard-to-reach" has been used to refer to certain segments of the audience that prove difficult to reach during public health campaigns (Hourani, Lambert, Peeler, Lane, & Borst, 2017). Freimuth and Mettger (1990) note that health communication campaigns are often mandated to reach target groups that have the highest risk, and when they fail, they label the groups as "hard-to-reach". As a reflection of the communicators' frustrations to reach people unlike themselves, these groups have been called obstinate, recalcitrant, chronically uninformed, disadvantaged, have-nots, illiterate, multifunctional, and information-poor (ibid.). People of low socioeconomic status and ethnic minorities have been labelled as hard-to-reach segments. Other hard-to-reach audiences are teenagers, people who do not speak the main languages used in the communication context (e.g. immigrants), chemically addicted persons, the homeless, the sick, and other vulnerable individuals. Hard-to-reach groups can be diverse, difficult to define, and purpose-dependent. Disengaged target groups can also fall under this category of hard-to-reach.

In the USA, for example, blacks, Native Americans, and Hispanic Americans are often labelled as hard-to-reach or hardly reached. Blacks and Hispanics have been labelled as hard-to-reach because their cultures are different from the mainstream culture (Freimuth & Mettger, 1990), a vivid reminder of the role of cultural aspects in health communication. Several explanations account for the challenges, including that their cultures are not understood by those who plan communication, language differences, especially with Hispanic audiences, history of racial relations (e.g. African Americans) and how it influences both the communicator and the recipients, low literacy levels, inadequate information processing skills, poor communication skills, limited access to communication channels, distrust of public institutions, and that their messages may not be adequately tailored for the groups (Freimuth & Mettger, 1990). These explanations are indicative of the cultural complexity of the rhetorical context. Pandemic communications in the USA, as in other parts of the world, are heavily shaped by past historical experiences and cultures.

The pandemic has highlighted the need for governments to timely reach all their citizens with risk information. In the context of infectious diseases, overseeing certain groups can diminish the objectives of risk communication and lead to far-reaching consequences for society as a whole. A good example can be drawn from the relatively homogenous Scandinavian countries: Denmark, Norway, and Sweden. In all three countries, it was clear that migrants were over-represented in most statistics relating to infections, hospitalization, and deaths (see Diaz et al., 2020). While there are many explanatory factors to the higher COVID-19 mortality and morbidity among migrant groups, such as poor social and living conditions in crowded neighbourhoods and work conditions, poor targeted communication was one of the contributory factors. While the governments in the Scandinavian countries devoted more time to providing COVID-19 information through frequent press conferences, extensive mainstream media coverage, and official websites, the information somehow eluded some of the migrant groups. Linguistic and cultural barriers prevented access to vital risk information, comprehension of messages, and compliance with recommendations. Another possible explanation is that migrant groups have access to other information from their home countries of origin. The likelihood of getting mixed and contradictory messages is higher compared to the rest of the population.

It is important to notice that migrant groups are also not homogeneous, and this is where the challenges begin. Understanding these audience groups (migrants) can be a mammoth task but can also be key in developing targeted messages. In Denmark, for example, the COVID-19-related information was translated into 19 different languages. As Diaz et al. (2020) note, "information was mainly translated using non-professional interpreters by non-governmental organizations (NGOs) with limited resources and qualifications, which to some extent compromised the timeliness and quality" (p. 2). The lack of professional medical interpreters compromised the quality of translations. Similar limitations were noted in Sweden and Norway where translations were barely adequate. There were other subgroups who the authorities failed to reach. In Norway, infection rates and hospitalizations were higher for migrants from Somalia, Pakistan, and Afghanistan and lower for migrants from Poland, Romania, and Lithuania in the first wave. Somali migrants were one of the subgroups that registered higher incidence rates in all three Scandinavian countries. It was evident that the Scandinavian countries lacked clear and visible strategies targeting specific migrant communities, especially in the first wave. The generalized strategies they employed left out other subgroups like the Somali communities. Brekke (2021) refers to some of these groups as "hard-to-reach immigrant groups", referring to the apparent failure of the Norwegian media to reach the Somali communities.

Another subgroup of immigrants that have been in the shadows of COVID-19 information is non-registered migrants. Many countries in Europe, Asia, the USA, and some African countries are host to unregistered and undocumented migrants. This migrant subgroup faces unique vulnerabilities compared to other migrant groups. In addition to other social challenges they face, they also have limited access to the healthcare system and will avoid contact with health authorities due to fears that their status would be exposed to authorities. They will prefer to remain invisible rather than face possible arrests or deportation. This deters them from seeking care when sick, testing, or vaccination. Contact tracing is also hampered because very often these groups have little encounter with government institutions. Burton-Jeangros et al. (2020) note that undocumented migrants are at an even higher risk of adverse consequences during a crisis due to a lack of access to essential securities and sources of support. They face particular challenges related to access to information. Understanding the specific communication needs of this "hard-to-reach" or hardly reached group can help authorities find alternative strategies to reach them with information.

How to Overcome Obstacles with "Hard-to-Reach" Audiences

How best can public health authorities reach out to the so-called hard-to-reach audiences? What experiences can we draw from the pandemic? The starting point is to understand the reasons why certain audiences are difficult to reach. Most of the reasons are articulated above, especially the cultural aspects of the audiences and the mainstream cultures. Froonjian and Garnett (2013) note that public officials lack access to certain groups due to the following factors:

- Language barriers
- Distrust of government or service providers
- Lack of attendance at government meetings
- No access to mainstream government mailings, postings, e-mails, or advertising
- A dangerous or isolated physical environment
- Lack of transportation
- Lack of government resources to expand communication efforts

Understanding the communication challenges will enable communicators to devise better strategies and plans.

Another strategy is underpinned in Freimuth and Mettger's (1990) search for alternative conceptualizations that move away from pejorative labels and preconceptions of viewing "hard-to-reach" audiences as powerless, apathetic, and isolated to more nuanced approaches in which individuals are seen as members of equivalent, albeit different, cultures. The label has negative connotations for those targeted because it implies that they have a deficit and are more difficult to communicate with than other audiences. Freimuth and Mettger build on the ideas of Ettema and Kline (1977) who emphasize the need for emphasising difference rather than deficit. Hard-to-reach audiences should not be viewed as having a deficit when compared to the mainstream dominant culture. They have differences rather than deficits. Ettema and Kline argue that when people are motivated to acquire information and that information is functional in their lives, they will make use of it. However, it is a widely accepted view among researchers that certain population segments require special efforts and strategies for communication (Froonjian & Garnett, 2013). The pandemic showed that some audiences have characteristics that make them hard to reach and governments have to adapt new strategies to communicate with them. The following sections explore some of the strategies used to overcome the barriers.

Communication-as-dialogue Approach

Researchers have looked at the conceptualization of the communication process and the perceptions of audiences. A conventional concept of the public communication campaign is based on a set of assumptions about the communicator, the message, and the audience. As Dervin (1989) notes, audiences are often seen as people to whom messages are to be transmitted artfully well, given their elusiveness. The conceptualization presupposes a one-way flow of communication, with efforts directed at targeting messages. Dervin (1989) criticizes these assumptions and proposes alternative conceptualizations of the communication process. She proposes a sense-making approach that allows audiences to make sense of their everyday life. Sense-making emphasize the need to listen to the audiences – how they see their situations: past, present, and future – and how they make sense and meaning of their situation (Dervin, 1989). Building further on this theory, Dervin and Frenette (2001) call for a dialogical campaign design that views audiences as listeners and learners who should be engaged dialogically. This approach ensures that audiences are not only heard but also have their perspectives acted upon. The approach emphasizes a two-way communication process.

More recently, there has been a shift in the understanding of risk communication from merely a one-way communication flow to an emphasis on a two-way communication process involving sharing of information and promoting dialogue between technical experts and stakeholders (Ndlela, 2019). Recent conceptualizations of risk communication emphasize the aspect of dialogue. Risk communication is conceived as a two-way process of communication, placing value on the quality of dialogue between experts and non-experts. Dialogue eliminates asymmetrical forms of relationships, inclining more towards mutual understanding. In an ideal situation, risk communication should function as a dialogue between governments, health authorities, and all other relevant stakeholders. As Sellnow and Sellnow (2010) note, dialogue cannot be achieved without credibility and trust. Researchers in communication have identified source credibility as a mitigating variable in risk communication. Factors affecting perceptions of credibility are "openness, accuracy, trustworthiness, impartiality and completeness of the information provided to the citizens" (McComas, 2003). Trust revolves around perceptions of persons or agencies as "competent, objective, fair, consistent, having no hidden agenda" (Heath, Seshadri, & Lee, 1998).

Sandman (1989) argues that the principle of involving the public in risk issues, whether it is risk assessment, decision-making, management, or communication, is crucial. Dialogue-based risk communication aims to bring together diverse stakeholders in risk knowledge creation and sharing. This approach recognizes that certain risks are complex and multidisciplinary; hence, they need to be addressed through dialogue with and participation by diverse stakeholders. Increasing stakeholder participation raises the likelihood of the message being credible. There is a growing realization by risk researchers that for risk communication to be effective, it should have a stakeholder perspective. Dialogue-based perspectives are captured in the definition of risk communication by Lang et al. (2001): "[R]isk communication is any purposeful exchange of information about risks between interested parties". In their "General Principles of Food Safety Risk Management", the World Health Organization (WHO) and the FAO (Food and Agriculture Organization) hold that "risk management should include clear, interactive communication with consumers and other interested parties in all aspects of the process". In its project to investigate what type of communication would improve the public understanding of flood risk and encourage people to take action, the British Environment Agency (2015) carried out a major public dialogue project on flood risk communication. In its project evaluation, it found that "getting people and communities involved in talking about flood risks increase people's understanding of local flood risk and can help them on a journey towards making preparations to protect themselves against flooding" (Environment Agency, 2015). Properly applied dialogue-based risk communication can help stakeholders and experts share knowledge and understanding of the risk issue. Dialogue is aimed at ensuring that a diverse range of people share a common understanding of the risk issue with the organizations/individuals in charge of managing the risk concerned.

The pandemic severely tested the leadership abilities to get other stakeholders on board. It also highlighted why open and honest dialogue was necessary to get important stakeholders to accept the government's intrusive measures. Governments had to engage in dialogue with different private sector organizations, private businesses, religious organizations, and so forth. Guiding a crisis response nationally required extensive participation of key societal actors, including the public. In their research on COVID-19 response in New Zealand, McGuire et al. (2020) examine the use of different mediums, such as parliamentary statements, daily briefings, Facebook Live broadcasts, and podcasts as mechanisms for engaging in direct dialogue with the public. Despite the challenges of engaging in dialogue with the public, there are idealistic reasons for engaging the population. In democratic societies, engaging and hearing the voice of all people is one of the fundamental cornerstones. Governments in democratic societies are obliged to engage with their citizens through all available means of communication.

In a crisis, public authorities should endeavour to interact with target groups, including those that are deemed hard-to-reach. Public administrators should be able to interact with groups that cannot be reached through mainstream communication channels (Froonjian & Garnett, 2013) and engage in dialogue rather than simply send information, which often results in a one-way communication flow (Freimuth & Mettger, 1990).

Reaching Distrustful Audiences via Trusted Communicators

Research and best practices highlight the value of using trusted individuals as intermediaries between public authorities and hard-to-reach audiences. Lack of trust in public authorities has been recognized as one of the factors contributing to the barriers to communicating with hard-to-reach audience. In this environment, well-meaning messages from the authorities can be misconstrued or rejected, consequentially leading to harm that could have been avoided. Newspapers, mass media, and town hall meetings are increasingly ineffective in reaching people who may be linguistically isolated or distrustful of the government (Froonjian & Garnett, 2013). Communicators still have to find other means of reaching hard-to-reach audiences. Paul Lazarfled's two-step flow theory provides a framework for the flow of information from authorities to the audience via trusted individuals (opinion leaders). In the wake of the pandemic, authorities in different settings used opinion leaders in their quest to reach hard-to-reach target groups. Efforts included targeting specific population groups and establishing a partnership with grassroots opinion leaders.

For example, in Norway, national and local authorities adjusted their general strategies to incorporate intermediaries from immigrant communities and other hard-to-reach groups. In light of the over-representation of the Somali groups in COVID-19 statistics, Oslo authorities turned to other strategies to reach out to the migrant communities, including direct contact with immigrant youths, posters, and visits to the immigrant shops. One district in Oslo realized a need for a different strategy specifically for the Somali community. They turned to "information ambassadors" drawn from the Somali community. "The idea was to secure information to the Somali community by applying a bottom-up instead of a top-down approach and using members of the community as volunteer expert communicators" (Brekke, 2021, p. 10). Using structures like local mosques, they recruited representatives from the community to disseminate COVID-19 information. The messenger had to be people trusted by the Somali communities and the channels of communication and language had to resonate with the audiences. Brekke's case studies illustrate the limitations of traditional communication strategies in reaching out to certain migrant groups. The challenges of migrant audiences are not unique to Scandinavia. Similar challenges were observed in other countries. In a crisis like a pandemic, public authorities should realize the individuality of different groups and make sure communication is tailored to true members of the group (Brackertz et al., 2005) and that messages are conveyed by trusted members of the target communities in formats that are culturally congruent.

Reaching Hard-to-Reach Audiences through Influencers

Hard-to-reach target groups can be reached through intermediaries such as macro-, micro-, and nano influencers. Macro-influencers have many followers (e.g. more than 100,000), micro-influencers have a moderate number of followers (e.g. between 10,000 and 100,000), and nano influencers have between 1,000 and 10,000. In this communication landscape, the power has shifted, and some individuals have thousands and even millions of followers, listeners, and viewers. During a pandemic, influencers reached millions of their followers with pandemic-related messages, some reinforcing government messages, but some of which were not in lieu of official positions of the scientific community. Some influencers added weight to unsubstantiated claims, false news, and conspiracy theories. One can sit in one corner of the world and still manage to influence millions of followers, miles away and across geographical boundaries. A good illustration of the power of influencers during a crisis is Donald Trump's use of Twitter during his presidency. His tweets attracted a worldwide audience, including international media. The White House recognized Trump's tweets as official statements (Landers, 2017). However, Trump has been accused of spreading misinformation about the COVID-19 virus, thereby undermining the authority of institutions like the Centers for Disease Control and Prevention (CDC). One such example is his endorsement of unproved therapies such as hydroxychloroquine and chloroquine as potential medication against the novel COVID-19 disease. Niburski and Niburski (2020) have studied the impact of Trump's promotion of unproven COVID-19 treatments. They note that Trump's tweets touting hydroxychloroquine and chloroquine as potential cures generated at least 2% of airtime in mainstream conservative media networks in the USA and increased Google searches and purchases. For example, purchases of medicine substitutes such as hydroxychloroquine increased by 200% in Amazon (ibid.). Niburski and Niburski (2020) conclude that "individuals in positions of power can sway public purchasing, resulting in undesired effects when the individuals' claims are unverified".

A countless number of influencers have played different roles in the pandemic information landscape, sharing health news of diverse sorts – useful healthy advice, educational messages, but also humour, fake news, satire, misinformation, and conspiracy theories around the coronavirus. Some influencers have voiced their support or opposition to vaccinations and other guidelines promoted by the public authorities. A report by the Center for Countering Digital Hate (CCDH) (2021), "The Disinformation Dozen", found that the modern anti-vaccination movement was spearheaded by a relatively small number of influencers. These were well-devoted and well-financed individuals who accounted for more than 65% of anti-vaccine content. CCDH noted that while many people might spread anti-vaccine content on their social media, much of this information emanated from just a few influencers. These anti-vaccine influencers reached many social media users around the world, essentially influencing their risk perception and aversion to recommendations from health authorities. The influence of such information was self-evident in the number of people resisting or reluctant to take vaccinations.

Some influencers have however used their power positively to support official public communications. Some were formally co-opted by governments and organizations to spread information in their circles. Abidin et al. (2021) note how some governments formally enlisted the help of influencers to manage the information landscape. They cite the example of Finland, the UK and Indonesia. In Finland, the government classified social media influencers as critical actors in society during a crisis, along with doctors, bus drivers, and grocery store workers (Heikkila, 2020). In the UK, the government enlisted influencers to help spread accurate messages to younger audiences. This was part of the government's efforts to combat misinformation circulated mainly via social media. Young people were most exposed to misinformation because they got most of their information through social media. As Pritchard (2020) notes, the UK government set aside funds for organizations like the Humanitarian-to-Humanitarian (H2H) Network for fact-fighting work and for the use of influencers to help spread accurate information about the coronavirus. This endeavour sought to reach young people in East Asia and Africa.

It is therefore important for communicators to revisit the role of influencers during a public health crisis. Some influencers can constitute a vital asset for reaching audiences with crucial public health messages. In the past, governments were able to communicate with the public through the mass media like television, but nowadays younger people access their news via social media. Unlike governments, social media influencers have huge access to the audience and influence in their circles. The Finnish example shows how social media influencers can be harnessed for the good of crisis communication by helping to get the message across.

Conclusion

Audiences are a central puzzle in risk and crisis communication where lives are threatened. Communicators are obliged to communicate with as many people as possible. Many challenges of public communication hinge on the audience and many of the failures in communication stem from misconceptions about the audiences. Drawing lessons from research and practice, communicators can effectively communicate risk and crisis messages. Research and practitioners alike concur that understanding your audience is the most important factor in effective communication (Freberg, 2019; T. L. Sellnow & Seeger, 2021; Sutherland, 2021). Audiences have diverse backgrounds and contexts that impact on the understanding of risk and risk aversion behaviours. Knowledge about the audiences, both intended and unintended audiences, forms the basis for effective communication. This presupposes that the communicator identifies target audiences and seeks information about them. More importantly, the communicator should seek interaction with the target audiences, enhance chances for dialogical communication to supplement one-way flows, form partnerships with actors and individuals that interact with target audiences, and gain trust or filter messages through trusted individuals. As Garnett (1992) aptly puts it, communicating through sources credible to a target audience improves odds of reaching that audience. Understanding audiences is very crucial in any risk communication. Segmenting the audiences into clear categories allows for the tailoring of communication strategies, selection of correct communication channels, and crafting of appropriate messages. During the crisis, taking into account the diversity of audience groups and providing each with relevant, timely, and accurate information about the unfolding crisis is a crucial step in resolving the crisis.

References

Abidin, C., Lee, J., Barbetta, T., & Miao, W. S. (2021). Influencers and COVID-19: Reviewing key issues in press coverage across Australia, China, Japan, and South Korea. *Media International Australia, 178*(1), 114–135. doi:10.1177/1329878x20959838

Anderson, R. M., Heesterbeek, H., Klinkenberg, D., & Hollingsworth, T. D. (2020). How will country-based mitigation measures influence the course of the COVID-19 epidemic? *Lancet, 395*(10228), 931–934. doi:10.1016/s0140-6736(20)30567-5

Blanchard-Boehm, R. D. (1998). Understanding public response to increased risk from natural hazards: Application of the hazards risk communication framework. *International Journal of Mass Emergencies Disasters, 16*, 247–278.

Brackertz, N., Zwart, I., Meredyth, D., & Ralston, L. (2005). Community consultation and the 'hard to reach' concepts and practice in Victorian local government. Swinburne, Australia. Retrieved from https://apo.org.au/sites/default/files/resource-files/2005-12/apo-nid2800.pdf

Brekke, J.-P. (2021). Informing hard-to-reach immigrant groups about COVID-19—Reaching the Somali population in Oslo. *Journal of Refugee Studies, 35*(1), 641–661. doi:10.1093/jrs/feab053

Burton-Jeangros, C., Duvoisin, A., Lachat, S., Consoli, L., Fakhoury, J., & Jackson, Y. (2020). The impact of the Covid-19 pandemic and the lockdown on the health and living conditions of undocumented migrants and migrants undergoing legal status regularization. *Frontiers in Public Health, 8*. doi:10.3389/fpubh.2020.596887

Center for Countering Digital Hate. (2021). The disinformation dozen: Why platforms must act on twelve leading online anti-vaxxers. Retrieved from https://counterhate.com/research/the-disinformation-dozen/#about

Chen, C., Frey, C. B., & Presidente, G. (2021). Culture and contagion: Individualism and compliance with COVID-19 policy. *Journal of Economic Behavior & Organization, 190*, 191–200. doi:10.1016/j.jebo.2021.07.026

Cialdini, R. B., & Goldstein, N. J. (2004). Social influence: Compliance and conformity. *Annual Review of Psychology, 55*, 591–621. doi:10.1146/annurev.psych.55.090902.142015

Dervin, B. (1989). Audience as listener and learner, teacher and confidante: The sense-making approach. In R. Rice, E & C. K. Atkin (Eds.), *Public Communication Campaigns* (2 ed., pp. 67–86). Newbury Park, CA: Sage Publications.

Dervin, B., & Frenette, M. (2001). Sensemaking methodology: Communicating communicatives with campaign audiences. In R. Rice, E. & C. K. Atkin (Eds.), *Public Communication Campaigns* (3 ed., pp. 69–87). London: Sage Publications.

Diaz, E., Norredam, M., Aradhya, S., Benfield, T., Krasnik, A., Madar, A., & Juarez, S. (2020). Situational brief: Migration and Covid-19 in Scandinavian countries. Retrieved from https://migrationhealth.org/wp-content/uploads/2021/05/lancet-migration-situational-brief-skandinavia-01-en.pdf

Environment Agency. (2015). *Public Dialogues on Flood Risk Communication* (SC120010/R1). Retrieved from https://www.gov.uk/flood-and-coastal-erosion-risk-management-research-reports/public-dialogues-on-flood-risk-communication (Accessed 21.06.2023).

Ettema, J. S., & Kline, F. G. (1977). Deficits, differences, and ceilings: Contingent conditions for understanding the knowledge gap. *Communication Research, 4*(2), 179–202. doi:10.1177/009365027700400204

Frandsen, F., & Johansen, W. (2017). *Organizational Crisis Communication.* Los Angeles, CA: Sage.

Freberg, K. (2019). *Social Media for Strategic Communication.* Los Angeles: Sage.

Freimuth, V., Linnan, H., W., & Potter, P. (2000). Communicating the threat of emerging infections to the public. *Emerging Infectious Diseases, 6*(4), 337–347.

Freimuth, V., & Mettger, W. (1990). Is there a hard-to-reach audience? *Public Health Reports, 105*(3), 232–238.

Froonjian, J., & Garnett, J. L. (2013). Reaching the hard to reach: Drawing lessons from research and practice. *International Journal of Public Administration, 36*(12), 831–839. doi:10.1080/01900692.2013.795161

Fuchs, C. (2021). *Communicating Covid-19.* London: Emerald Publishing.

Garnett, J. L. (1992). *Communicating for Results in Government: A Strategic Approach for Public Managers.* San Francisco, CA: Jossey-Bass.

Gelfand, M. J., Jackson, J. C., Pan, X., Nau, D., Pieper, D., Denison, E., . . . Wang, M. (2021). The relationship between cultural tightness–looseness and COVID-19 cases and deaths: A global analysis. *The Lancet Planetary Health, 5*(3), e135–e144. doi:10.1016/S2542-5196(20)30301-6

Gelfand, M. J., Raver, J. L., Nishii, L., Leslie, L. M., Lun, J., Lim, B. C., . . . Yamaguchi, S. (2011). Differences between tight and loose cultures: A 33-nation study. *Science, 332*(6033), 1100–1104. doi:10.1126/science.1197754

Gupta, M., Shoja, A., & Mikalef, P. (2022). Toward the understanding of national culture in the success of non-pharmaceutical technological interventions in mitigating COVID-19 pandemic. *Annals of Operations Research, 319*(1), 1433–1450. doi:10.1007/s10479-021-03962-z

Heath, R. L., Seshadri, S., & Lee, J. (1998). Risk communication: A two-community analysis of proximity, dread, trust, involvement, uncertainty, openness/accessibility, and knowledge on support/opposition toward chemical companies. *Journal of Public Relations Research, 10*(1), 35–56. doi:10.1207/s1532754xjprr1001_02

Heikkila, M. (2020). Finland taps social media influencers during coronavirus crisis. Retrieved from https://www.politico.eu/article/finland-taps-influencers-as-critical-actors-amid-coronavirus-pandemic/

Hofstede, G. (2001). *Culture's Consequences: Comparing Values, Behaviors, Institutions and Organizations across Nations* (2 ed.). London: Sage Publications.

Hourani, L., Lambert, S., Peeler, R., Lane, B., & Borst, C. (2017). Graphic novels: A new stress mitigation tool for military training: developing content for hard-to-reach audiences. *Health Communication, 32*(5), 541–549. doi:10.1080/10410236.2016.1140265

Huynh, T. L. D. (2020). Does culture matter social distancing under the COVID-19 pandemic? *Safety Science, 130*, 104872. doi:10.1016/j.ssci.2020.104872

Landers, E. (2017). White house: Trump's tweets are 'official statements'. Retrieved from https://edition.cnn.com/2017/06/06/politics/trump-tweets-official-statements/index.html

Lang, S., Fewtrell, L., & Bartram, J. (2001). Risk communication. In W. H. O. (WHO) (Ed.), *Water Quality. Guidelines, Standards and Health: Assessment of Risk and Risk Management for Water-related Infectious Disease*. London: IWA Publishing.

McComas, K. A. (2003). Citizen satisfaction with public meetings used for risk communication. *Journal of Applied Communication Research, 31*(2), 164–184. doi:10.1080/0090988032000064605

McGuire, D., Cunningham, J. E. A., Reynolds, K., & Matthews-Smith, G. (2020). Beating the virus: An examination of the crisis communication approach taken by New Zealand Prime Minister Jacinda Ardern during the Covid-19 pandemic. *Human Resource Development International, 23*(4), 361–379. doi:10.1080/13678868.2020.1779543

Nair, N., Selvaraj, P., & Nambudiri, R. (2022). Culture and COVID-19: Impact of cross-cultural dimensions on behavioral responses. *Collection Encyclopedia of COVID-19, 2*(3), 1210–1224. Retrieved from https://www.mdpi.com/2673-8392/2/3/81

Ndlela, M. (2019). *Crisis Communication. A Stakeholder Perspective*. Cham: Switzerland: Palgrave Macmillan.

Niburski, K., & Niburski, O. (2020). Impact of Trump's promotion of unproven COVID-19 treatments and subsequent internet trends: Observational study. *Journal of Medical Internet Research, 22*(11), e20044–e20044. doi:10.2196/20044

Pritchard, T. (2020). The UK government's enlisted influencers to try and tackle coronavirus misinformation. Retrieved from https://www.gizmodo.com.au/2020/03/the-uk-governments-enlisted-influencers-to-try-and-tackle-coronavirus-misinformation/

Sandman, P. M. (1989). Hazard versus outrage in the public perception of risk. In V. T. Covello, D. B. McCallum, & M. T. Pavlova (Eds.), *Effective Risk Communication: The Role and Responsibility of Government and Nongovernment Organizations* (pp. 45–49). Boston, MA: Springer US.

Sellnow, T. L., & Seeger, M. W. (2021). *Theorizing Crisis Communication* (2 ed.). Hoboken, NJ: Wiley-Blackwell.

Sellnow, T., & Sellnow, D. D. (2010). The instructional dynamic of risk and crisis communication: Distinguishing instructional messages from dialogue. *Review of Communication, 10*(2), 112–126. doi:10.1080/15358590903402200

Sutherland, K. E. (2021). *Strategic Social Media Management: Theory and Practice*. Singapore: Palgrave Macmillan.

Triandis, H. C. (1989). The self and social behavior in differing cultural contexts. *Psychological Review, 96*(3), 506–520. doi:10.1037/0033-295X.96.3.506

9   Public Trust

Introduction

Countries around the world have had varying rates of COVID-19 infections and fatalities and rates of compliance with pandemic containment measures. While there are many contextual factors behind the variations, one of the factors cited by researchers and practitioners alike is the element of trust in the pandemic leadership, public authorities, and the media. In a study using data from 177 countries, Bollyky et al. (2022) concluded that trust in the government and in the people around correlated with lower COVID-19 infection rates. Levels of trust in the government and interpersonal trust had an impact on infection rates. Adamecz-Völgyi and Szabó-Morvai (2021) also found that "confidence in public institutions is one of the most important predictors of deaths attributed to COVID-19, compared to country-level measures of individual health risks, the health system, demographics, economic and political development, and social capital". In a pandemic, it matters how people react to containment measures, whether they obey or disobey stringent rules, comply with recommendations, for example, self-isolate or report being sick to authorities. People must have trust and confidence in their national authorities to be willing to comply. During the pandemic, public health communicators in many countries had to contend with diminishing public trust in state institutions and the mass media. Despite the many opportunities offered by digital communication platforms for the dissemination of information, pandemic messages have been met with scepticism or even outright rejection by the public. The central argument for this chapter is that trust is crucial for the successful containment of a public health crisis. This chapter argues that trust in state institutions and the mass media positively influences people's willingness to comply with public health messages as well as adopt behaviours that reduce the threat of an infectious disease. However, a lack of trust diminishes the possibility of the public adhering to the messages. Establishing and developing trust before a crisis occurs is vital for dealing with future health crises. Research from previous public health outbreaks has also highlighted the significance of trust in public health campaigns.

DOI: 10.4324/9781003401827-9

Conceptualising Trust

Trust is a broad, multifaceted concept that is used widely in different settings and disciplines. It remains a complex phenomenon not easy to define as there are many dimensions to trust. Mayer et al. (1995) define trust as "the willingness of a party to be vulnerable to the actions of another party based on the expectation that the other will perform a particular action important to the trustor, irrespective of the ability to monitor or control that other party" (p. 712). This definition of trust involves a willingness to take a risk and to be vulnerable. The trustor must be aware of the risk involved. Without risk, there is no reason to trust (Grosser, 2016). Several factors affect the trust one party has for another and one of these is the traits of the trustor. Hence, some parties are more likely to trust than others (Mayer et al., 1995). These are the factors that define the trustworthiness of others. Trustworthiness is influenced by several factors, including the ability (skills and competencies), benevolence (want to do good), and integrity (Ibid.). Trust involves the trustor's perception that the trustee observes a set of acceptable principles (ibid.). The trustor's personal integrity and moral integrity will therefore influence the quality of trust. As such, the trustworthiness of the trustee is not fixed. It is susceptible to change.

Literature on trust has identified different dimensions of trust. One method of differentiation identifies two types of trust: interpersonal and institutional. Interpersonal trust is defined as an "outcome of interpersonal interactions that people can learn to make decisions about future interactions", and these are based on the individual's past experiences of similar interactions (Ward, 2017). Institutional trust is defined as "the expected utility of institutions performing satisfactorily" (Sheppard & Sherman, 1998, p. 31). Trust in the system is based on the expectation that the system functions correctly (Grosser, 2016). Political trust refers to "citizens' assessments of the core institutions of the polity and entails a positive evaluation of the most relevant attributes that make each political institution trustworthy, such as credibility, fairness, competence, transparency in its policy-making, and openness to competing views" (Zmerli, 2014). Political trust has implications for higher or lower levels of trust in public policy (Marien & Hooghe, 2011).

Need for Trust

Why is trust important for a public health response? The need for trust can be addressed at the macro and micro levels of the pandemic response. At the macro level are supranational organizations, nations, and international institutions responsible for the co-ordination of international responses to a health outbreak. At the micro level are national and regional institutions tackling the outbreak in their backgrounds. Responding to a public health crisis requires that various actors (organizations and public health authorities) at all levels and the public work together to resolve the crisis. "Working together often involves interdependence, and people must therefore depend on others in various ways to accomplish their personal and organizational goals" (Mayer et al., 1995, p. 710). The working of different systems, such as politics, economics, science, the media, and many other systems that characterize modern society, is essential for the management of pandemics. A lack of trust in any of the above points in the system would undermine the efforts to mitigate the effects of the pandemic. The lack of trust can be manifested when there is a lack of transparency and trust in the pandemic response. This underscores the need to develop and cultivate good trust levels in the pre-crisis stages. Good trust levels during a crisis such as the COVID-19 pandemic presents better opportunities for achieving the best possible outcomes. The effectiveness of public health interventions is dependent on trust in central areas of a public health response. The following sections examine three areas that have been challenged during the pandemic:

- Political leadership
- Public health institutions
- Media institutions

Public Trust in Political Leadership

Pandemic crisis leadership involves many responsibilities, including sense-making, decision-making, terminating, and learning (A. Boin, Hart, Stern, & Sundelius, 2005). It involves getting tasks accomplished, influencing people effectively, and inducing necessary change (Van Wart, 2003). To persuade people, to comply with recommendations and containment regulations, invoke issues of public trust or distrust of the pandemic leadership. Public health campaigns depend heavily on participation and compliance by the public. "Public trust leads to greater compliance with a wide range of public policies, such as public health responses" (OECD, 2021a). When citizens do not trust the authorities, interventions are bound to fail. Lack of trust minimizes the effectiveness of the leadership, thus compounding the damages. "Catastrophic disasters, require additional leadership capabilities because extreme events overwhelm local capabilities and damage emergency response systems themselves" (Kapucu & Van Wart, 2008). The response system requires that leaders at different levels of administration do their work effectively. Leadership makes an enormous difference in managing emergencies and catastrophic events (Boin et al., 2005; Kapucu & Van Wart, 2008). Political actors at all levels of administration – local, regional, and national – constitute the first line of defence, playing a critical role in crisis prevention, mitigation, preparation, response, and recovery (McLean & Ewart, 2020). The role of local government is to manage crises at the local level and crisis preparation and response rest with local municipalities, where crisis management committees comprise elected officials and public officials. Political roles are embedded in the crisis management system. The local government must co-ordinate horizontally and vertically with other levels of administration within and across sectors. Co-ordination and collaboration are critical in crisis management and so is trust among agencies and communities.

The type of leadership will vary according to context. In less democratic societies, leadership often dictates what the public should do, whereas in liberal democracies, the leadership has to act within the confines of the law, free press, and accountability structures. Public trust in political leadership is pertinent for the management of pandemics. Political trust refers to "a basic evaluative or affective orientation toward the government" (Miller, 1974). It refers to how the public perceives various objects of trust in the political system, be it national legislatures, judiciary, national and local governments, and political institutions or the political system as a whole. Political trust is hence a broad concept prone to wide or narrow exploitations. It can mean support for, mistrust of, or dissatisfaction with the current regime as a whole or some components of it. Trust in government is "the degree to which people perceive that government is producing outcomes consistent with their expectations" (Hetherington, 2005). Like any form of trust, trust in government is based on expectations about the future (Marcinkowski & Starke, 2018). There are many variables that citizens use to base their evaluations of political authorities, and these include processes of decision-making, individual freedoms, economic welfare, and security. Trust in government is not absolute; hence the degree of trust or distrust is dynamic and bound to vary, depending on the issues and the context. Distrust arises when the system is not performing according to expectations or when the legitimacy of the government is questioned. Bertsou (2019) notes that political distrust is "a relational attitude that reflects perceptions of untrustworthiness specific to the political system in its entirety or its components" (p. 220). The consequences of political trust and distrust are imminent in a pandemic where the outcomes are reliant on the interdependencies between the government and the public.

The pandemic situation called for public leadership, as the public expected the governments and public agencies to make critical decisions necessary to prevent or mitigate the effects of the pandemic. The public expected those in charge to provide direction even in the most difficult circumstances (Boin et al., 2005). Leadership is expected during extraordinary situations. As Boin et al. (2005) note, "if the incumbent elites fail to step forward, others might well seize the opportunity to fill the gap" (p. 8). The coronavirus pandemic placed significant pressure on political leadership around the world. It highlighted the significance of trust in crisis management, as trusted leaders found it easier to convince their citizens about the necessity for stringent pandemic containment rules. Lack of trust in political leadership undoubtedly undermined responses in some countries, where leaders struggled to convince their citizens.

Unfortunately, political distrust has become commonplace in many countries, democracies and non-democracies alike. For example, polls by the Pew

Research Center in the US show that public trust in government has been eroding and is now near historic lows. The number of Americans who believe that the government can be trusted to do the right thing "most of the time" is low (22%). The government in the US had enormous challenges convincing its citizens due to increased political polarization in the country.

From Ebola to COVID-19

One challenge noted in Africa's response to the COVID-19 pandemic has been the low levels of public trust in the political leadership. Repeated surveys and research in Africa show that many countries in the region suffer from low levels of trust in political institutions and political leadership. Previous outbreaks such as Ebola highlighted the negative consequences of public distrust of government officials (Richardson, McGinnis, & Frankfurter, 2019). When we recall the Ebola outbreaks in West Africa in 2014 and later outbreaks in the Democratic Republic of Congo, mistrust in political leadership and institutions central to the crisis management efforts dampened efforts to quickly bring the outbreak under control. During the Ebola crisis, people were reluctant to comply with government-mandated sanitation and social distancing protocols aimed at containing the outbreak (Blair, Morse, & Tsai, 2017). Some individuals blatantly refused to comply with government mandates to quarantine or to follow safe burial practices (Dhillon & Kelly, 2015). Journalists reported stories of people not taking their sick relatives to health centres, hiding infected relatives from health officials, conducting secret burial ceremonies, not reporting the sick to the authorities, and taking their sick relatives for alternative healing in religious and traditional settings. There were even reports of people attacking health personnel. During the outbreak of Ebola in the Democratic Republic of Congo, the public was so distrustful of the local authorities and suspicious of the healthcare workers to the extent of even attacking health workers resulting in fatal clashes. It is evident that during the Ebola crisis in West Africa, a lack of trust in formal institutions of the states hampered the attempts to rein in the Ebola outbreak and aggravated the situation.

Years later into the pandemic, political leadership in most African countries still register low levels of trust and few have invested in boosting that trust. In 2016, a survey by Studiebarometer in 2016 noted that across 36 countries in Africa, people expressed more trust in informal institutions such as religious and traditional leaders (72% and 61%, respectively) than in formal institutions of the state (Bratton & Gyimah-Boadi, 2016). Surveys in Angola during the pandemic show that people in that country trust religious leaders and traditional leaders more than elected leaders (Afrobarometer, 2022). Other surveys from Afrobarometer show that some countries have registered declining trust in institutions. In South Africa, trust in Members of Parliament (MPs), provincial premiers, local government councils, the ruling party, and opposition parties declined dramatically, making political leaders the least trusted public officials in the country (Chingwete, 2016). As South Africa grappled with a third wave of COVID-19 infections, trust in nearly all institutions was low and declining, with little trust in the president (38%), parliament (27%), traditional leaders (31%), provincial premier (27%), the local council (24%), and religious leaders (42%) (Moosa & Hofmeyr, 2021). Not surprisingly, the South African government faced immense challenges in trying to persuade its citizens to follow health guidelines and regulations to limit the spread of the disease.

In Africa's largest economy, Nigeria, political leadership also faced challenges of trust. As Ezeibe et al. (2020) note in the case of Nigeria, one of the countries with the highest level of citizen distrust of government officials, citizens' distrust of the government contributed to the spread of the diseases:

> Political distrust during the COVID-19 era in Nigeria manifests in non-compliance to government directives to mitigate the virus such as stay-at-home orders, inter-state travels, curfews, closure of public gatherings exceeding 50 persons, wearing of face masks and maintaining personal hygiene. Others include escape of patients from isolation centres, protests of patients in isolation centres.
>
> (Ezeibe et al., 2020)

Ezeibe et al. (2020) noted that 86% of the respondents distrusted government initiatives to mitigate the spread of COVID-19 in Nigeria. A major factor driving distrust was the high levels of corruption in the country. Another source of distrust of government was the inefficiency of government institutions and inequality in the distribution of COVID-19 material. The effects of political distrust were apparent in the public disregard for government mandates. The observation by Ezeibe et al. (2020) that "political distrust makes people celebrate when the virus kills a politician" resonates with cases elsewhere in Africa, where the citizens viewed the pandemic as an equalizer, with politicians testing their own medicine. In Zimbabwe, the citizens took to social media to celebrate the COVID-19-related deaths of senior politicians and the son of a senior politician. They blamed the government for the poor state of the public hospitals and inadequately paid health workers. As one commentator noted:

> For the first time, our politicians and senior government leaders are confronting the reality of the decay in our health system; over the past few years they would fly to South Africa, to China, to Malaysia for treatment, but right now they have to face the years of neglect of which they are the chief parties.
>
> (Moyo, 2021)

Citizens' distrust of the government poses a threat to pandemic communications because it contributes to limited compliance with government messages.

In countries where citizens lacked trust in the political system, political leadership struggled to convince the public to adhere to certain behaviours such as staying at home, mask-wearing, and vaccinating. Disobedience and disregard for government mandates were noted in many countries across the world. Undoubtedly, political distrust undermines crisis communication messages. The public will need to trust the government and trust that government officials have their best intentions, before complying with the messages.

Leveraging "Trust Capital"

For some countries, trust in political leadership has been an asset during the pandemic response. A survey across 22 OECD (Organization for Economic Co-Operation and Development) countries by OECD (2021a) showed an even split between those who trust their government and those who distrust it. In countries like Norway and Finland, over 60% of the population trusts their government. Public trust in institutions is cited as one of the key elements of a successful response to the COVID-19 pandemic in Finland (OECD, 2021b), Norway (OECD, 2022), and New Zealand (OECD, 2023). The surveys highlight the significance of "trust capital" in addressing the pandemic. Public trust helps political leadership to respond to challenges facing society, reduces transaction costs, and ensures higher levels of compliance with public policies. A "good standing before a crisis might enable a leader or government to ride it out successfully and even build public trust" (Arjen Boin, McConnell, & Hart, 2008). Higher levels of public trust undoubtedly yielded positive levels of public compliance.

Public Trust in Health Institutions

Public health institutions are at the forefront of the response and management of disease outbreaks. In health care and public health, a key element is a principal-agent relationship. In such as relationship, one person (the principal/public) gives another person (the agent/public health system) authority to make decisions on his or her behalf (Shore, 2003, p. 14). Public health authorities represent the science-led approach behind the mitigation messages about the nature of the virus and how the public can protect themselves against it. Trust in these institutions is essential during a pandemic. It is the essential ingredient for effective health communication. It creates the environment in which the communication of messages and eventually persuasion takes place. The public is bound to accept and comply with messages if they trust the public health authorities.

Trust and open communication are listed as important factors in public health communication. Interaction between the governments, public health authorities, and the public rely on trust. In a pandemic, the primary source of public health information is public health institutions like the World Health Organization (WHO) and national institutions like the US Centers for Disease Control and Prevention (CDC), Norwegian Institute of Public Health (Norway), Public Health Agency of Sweden (Sweden), Centre for Disease Control (Nigeria), the National Institute for Health Protection (UK), or the ministries of health. These health authorities are central to pandemic responses and trust in these institutions has a bearing on how well their messages are received by the public.

Trust in public health officials and the information they provide is essential for the public uptake of preventative strategies to reduce the transmission of COVID-19 (Henderson et al., 2020). The central argument is that for public interventions to be successful, the public should at the minimum trust public health officials, their messages, and the science upon which their messaging is based (Ward, 2017). In a context where there are many competing voices and many sources of information, the public must rely on credible sources, such as disease control authorities for health messages.

Public trust in these agencies has never been as important as they were during the pandemic, given their central role in the crisis, yet some of them were also embroiled in another crisis, "the crisis of trust". For example, a survey report by Pollard and Davis (2021) shows the declining trust in the US CDC during the COVID-19 pandemic. Ernest-Samuel and Uduma (2022a) discuss the lack of credibility of the Nigerian Centre for Disease Control, which has faced outrage over the discrepancies in its statistics. At the beginning of the pandemic, statistics were used by governments around the world to justify lockdowns. Compliance with lockdown messages presupposes that the public believes in the statistics of infections and hospitalization coming from these authorities. Public health authorities around the world have faced accusations of either understating or overstating COVID-19 statistics for other ulterior motives. Narratives in Africa have accused governments of under-reporting COVID-19-related deaths to hide their inefficiency or exaggerating the numbers in order to attract more international aid. Even for the most advanced countries, questions about what to trust and what to ignore arose, given a confusing flurry of figures, graphs, and projections surrounding the pandemic (Richardson & Spiegelhalter, 2020). Public health authorities that were perceived as lowly in trustworthiness found it difficult to convince the public during the outbreak.

In most African countries, convincing people of the seriousness of COVID-19 proved to be difficult due to low levels of trust in public health authorities. This is aptly captured by Osman Dar, a health expert with the London-based Chatham House, in an interview with Deutsche Welle: "people are likely to ask 'if we have HIV, tuberculosis and malaria killing hundreds of thousands of people and the government doesn't care, why are you suddenly so worried about this coronavirus infection'"? (Krippahl, 2020). Past experiences with poor public health service delivery create long-lasting perceptions that African governments do not care about public health and that underfunded public health institutions are not good enough. Trust in local public health institutions is further diminished by the fact that national political leaders often sought medical attention outside their own countries. Africa has one of the weakest health systems globally (Tessema et al., 2021), and hence health institutions are lowly perceived on the questions of preparedness and capabilities. The main impediments to public health systems in Africa include lack of availability, accessibility of health care, limited resources, equipment, and personnel. These poor conditions were further exacerbated by higher incidences of corruption, embezzlement of COVID-19 funds, and poor management of isolation and quarantine centres (AllAfrica, 2020).

Media reports in several countries write about incidences of people running away from isolation and quarantine centres. In their research, Ezeibe et al. (2020) found that political distrust in Nigeria induced suspected COVID-19 carriers to escape from isolation centres. Some people hid their loved ones with suspected symptoms, while others attacked healthcare givers in isolation centres. Other people resorted to alternative medicine for cures. Africa is not alone in this quagmire. For various reasons, people have been reported running away from poorly managed isolation centres and health institutions in several countries around the world. One recurrent reason for absconding is trust in health institutions. Geelani and Gupta (2020) report of people in India fleeing from quarantine facilities and posing a risk of spreading the virus to society. The main reasons cited are the poor conditions in isolation and quarantine centres and the "extreme lack of trust in the public health care system" (Daniyal, 2020). In the article "Coronavirus, Why are Indians running away from isolation wards?" Daniyal (2020) noted that with the poor state of the Indian public healthcare system, many Indians were looking with suspicion at the state's efforts to battle the COVID-19 disease, creating complications for health authorities to grapple with. Daniyal further writes that so low was the trust in public healthcare that Indians tried to avoid the public system even when private healthcare could not accommodate them. Weak public health infrastructure and lack of trust in health institutions created a detrimental context for the pandemic response.

Vaccination: The Problem of Trust

"The most important ingredient in all vaccines is trust" – this quote from Barry Bloom of the Harvard T.H. School of Public Health aptly captures the significance of trust in any vaccination programme (quoted in OECD, 2021c). The OECD policy document "Enhancing public trust in COVID-19 vaccination: The role of governments" stresses the importance of trust in the vaccination programmes when it alludes that "public trust in COVID-19 vaccines and vaccination will be as essential as the vaccines themselves" (OECD, 2021c). Before taking a vaccination, people seek information about the vaccines, the vaccination types, the science behind them, their safety, how they would be handled and administered, and the overall risk factors linked to them. As such, trust is essential in any vaccination programme, where both the vaccination and the governments are put to test. The uptake of vaccination depends on the ability of governments to convince the public about the benefits and safety of vaccinations. Citizens who trust their governments, public health authorities, and political leadership are willing to listen and likely comply, whereas citizens who do not trust their governments are likely to hesitate. The OECD policy report states that trust in vaccination and in the ability of the governments to communicate and to successfully implement the vaccination programme are critically dependent on:

- Public confidence in the effectiveness and safety of the vaccines
- The competence and reliability of the institutions to deliver them
- Principles and processes guiding government decisions and action (i.e. vaccine procurement and distribution)
- The capacity and effectiveness of regulatory agencies
- Public engagement and communications

(OECD, 2021c)

The issues of trust mentioned above have a bearing on all vaccination programmes. Institutions that have earned trust before the crisis have a better starting point and leverage than those with low levels of trust. Governments with low trust have the daunting task of trying to earn the trust of their citizens and at the same time, trying to promote the vaccine.

One of the most controversial areas in the response to the COVID-19 pandemic has centred around perceptions of vaccinations. Across the world, hesitancy towards vaccination has been recorded, and much of this is related to trust or lack of trust in governments, public health authorities, and pharmaceuticals. The lack of trust in these critical institutions undoubtedly had negative impacts on the people's willingness to be vaccinated. Even while health officials expressed the urgent need to get people vaccinated against the virus, several obstacles lay in the way as the governments ran into the problem of trust.

In Africa, most governments quickly ran into the problem of trust: trust in governments and trust in vaccines. In a survey by Afrobarometer in five West African countries of Benin, Liberia, Niger, Senegal, and Togo, only three in ten citizens (31%) said that they trusted their government to ensure that any vaccine was safe (Seydou, 2021). Mistrust was directed to the government's capacity to not only choose the right types of vaccines but also to handle and administer them safely. The survey highlighted a strong correlation between trust in government and the likelihood to get vaccinated (Figure 9.1).

Some people would rather opt for traditional herbs or pray instead of taking a vaccine (ibid.). Findings from national surveys in 34 African countries indicate that "almost six out of 10 respondents (58%) said they believe that prayer was 'somewhat more effective' or 'much more effective' than a vaccine in preventing COVID-19 infection" (Katenda, 2022). The conspiracy theories flourishing in social media also added to the low levels of trust in government, health institutions, and vaccines. A survey of COVID-19 vaccine acceptance across

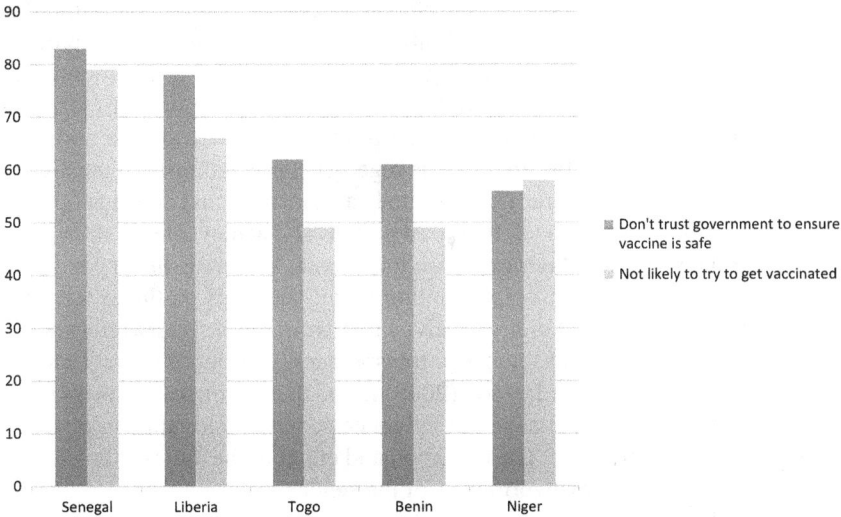

Figure 9.1 Trust on government and likelihood to get vaccinated.
Source: Afrobarometer.

23 countries in 2022 by Lazarus et al. (2023) found that vaccine hesitancy remained substantial around the world, partly due to the proliferation of misinformation. While vaccinations have been seen as a cornerstone of the pandemic response, public support remains elusive due to various reasons, including the low levels of trust. Most researchers concur that trust in public authorities increases the acceptance of vaccinations, while lack of trust, however, leads to vaccine hesitancy or rejection (Ward, Attwell, Meyer, Rokkas, & Leask, 2017).

Trust in Messengers

Trust in messengers is a critical element in risk and crisis communication that has a profound influence on how individuals respond to public health messages. Trust in the source of the message is crucial for persuasion and acceptance by the audience. Most researchers concur that people comply with messages only when they trust the messenger (Arriola & Grossman, 2021; Demeshko et al., 2022). As Seydou (2021) aptly puts it, "people are less likely to comply with public health messages if they do not trust the messenger". When the public trust the spokesperson (the messenger), they are more likely to change their opinion than with a spokesperson they do not trust (Hovland & Weiss, 1951). The WHO identifies that selecting "the best" spokesperson (or messenger) is important to ensure that communications are trusted (WHO, 2017). The authority and credibility of the source will make a big difference in how well a message is received by the audience. If the public perceives the messenger as a credible person, they are more likely to be persuaded. Credibility is "judgements made by a perceiver (e.g. a message recipient) concerning the believability of a communicator" (O'Keefe, 2002, p. 181). Source credibility affects the reception of messages. To be credible, the source should be well informed, knowledgeable about the subject, have expertise in the area, and is regarded as an authority in the area.

The reputation of the source (e.g. public health institutions) depends on what the audience knows about them, their past actions and achievements, their experience over the years, and their expertise in the area. In a crisis like a pandemic, the credibility of public health information largely depends on the expertise of the source of messages and their perceived trustworthiness. Trustworthiness includes such characteristics as honesty, transparency, just, morality, and ethical. In their work, Tormala and Clarkson (2008) found that the trustworthiness of the source of an early (prior) message can influence people's motivation to process a subsequent (target) message. The reception and effect of the message are closely linked to the perceived trustworthiness of the sender.

The COVID-19 pandemic demonstrated the need for trusted messengers, be it government spokespersons, or influential messengers like opinion leaders (i.e. influencers, religious leaders, and traditional leaders). However, it should be noted that a trusted source in one context is not necessarily trusted in other contexts. Hence, understanding the context of communication is vital in selecting appropriate spokespersons and messengers. The trustworthiness of the messenger is one of the most important factors that determine the success of healthy communication messages and public compliance. Research from Nigeria showed distrust of information emanating from the Nigerian authorities by the public (Adeitan, Onyechi, & Omah, 2021). If receivers perceive the messenger as untrustworthy, they are bound to seek other sources of information and public health communication is curtailed: "While searching between channels, they decide what information they trust, the credibility of the source and how the information provided by each source applies to them" (McLean & Ewart, 2020, p. 50). In the age of digital communications and social media, such sources are endless. Many other voices have messages to convey to whoever believes in them. People seek out and encounter information from sources they trust. The issue of who delivers the message is equally important as the message itself. Lack of trust in the spokesperson arguably diminishes the possibility of the public adhering to the messages such as restrictions on movement.

Trust in Media

The media have a special role to play in society, serving as conduits of information, news, opinions, education, and entertainment. They keep citizens informed about what is going on in their society, set agendas, and thereby influence public opinions regarding various issues. Media also act as watchdogs, reporting on the malpractices in society and raising public awareness. In a way, the media shape society in various ways. The media have a pivotal role to play during a public health crisis, providing information to the public who need it most. During a pandemic crisis, where stakes and risks to lives are high, authorities rely on the media to quickly disseminate vital information to the public. Authorities need the media to help their audiences understand the nature of the virus and advice on what they should do to avoid harm and protect their lives. Public authorities use the media to reach target audiences through press conferences, news releases, and other media appearances. The media, through news reports, debate, comment, and interpret the crisis. The perspective they take to frame the crisis influence public perceptions of the crisis and also those managing the crisis. As such, the media constitute a key element in the containment of a public health crisis. Access to reliable information is crucial during a public health crisis, not only to keep the public informed but to provide instructional messages on safety and health.

During the COVID-19 pandemic, media disseminated risk-related news and provided updates on health risk knowledge and other vital statistics (e.g. infections, hospitalization, recovery, and deaths). The media played an indispensable role during the pandemic. Yet, there have been concerns on the issue of public trust in the media institution and the influences on people's willingness to comply with public health messages as well as adopting behaviours that reduce the threat of an infectious disease. While research shows that during a crisis people turn to the public media for information about the pending crisis, several polls have shown a declining public trust in the media in many countries around the world. The 2021 Edelman's Trust Barometer shows an increased public mistrust of journalists in 28 countries. In the UK, despite the public relying on the news media as primary sources, journalists were the least trusted source of information regarding the pandemic, with 43% of the surveyed trusting them to report the truth, a figure lower than trust on government officials (48%) (ibid.). The Edelman's Trust Barometer results are similar to the findings from surveys conducted by the Reuter Institute for the Study of Journalism (Newman, Fletcher, Robertson, Eddy, & Nielsen, 2022).

Surveys by the Reuters Institute show that trust in the news has declined in many parts of the world and many continue to regard the news with considerable scepticism (Toff et al., 2021). The Reuters Institute Digital News Report survey across 18 countries shows that trust in the news media has fallen by an average of 5% (Fletcher, 2020). In their research on the UK media system, Mansell et al. (2019) note that "established practices of journalistic verification, institutional accountability and ethical 'truth filters' of a free, but responsible, news media are being dismantled" (p. 7). They identify five areas of the information crisis: *confusion* (citizens are less sure about what is true and whom to believe); *cynicism* (citizens are losing trust, even in trustworthy sources); *fragmentation* (citizens have access to many sources of information); *irresponsibility* (power over meaning is held by organizations that lack a developed ethical code of responsibility); and *apathy* (citizens disengage from established structures of society). The combination of these factors is a threat to, among others, individual decision-making.

The trust between the media and authorities is also fragile, leading to situations where authorities gauged the media during the pandemic. While the media are central to the resolution of the crisis, they can also constitute a crisis through sensationalising, dramatising, or peddling fear-arousing messages about the crisis or even undermining the narratives of crisis managers. To prevent the media from carrying alternative narratives, some countries put restrictions on COVID-19 reporting. They put measures or legislation restricting access to information and certain places. These restrictions were justified on sanitary requirements (social distancing) or prevention of disinformation. A report by Reporters Without Borders (RSF) shows a dramatic deterioration of press freedom during the pandemic in almost three-quarters of the world (Reporters Without Borders, 2021). It notes an increase in obstacles to news coverage and blocking of access to information reporting in the field. Countries, including Turkey, Hungary, Philippines, Russia, Saudi Arabia, and Malaysia, introduced new legislation or amended existing laws as part of the measures to combat disinformation (Holt, 2021). The laws criminalized publishing so-called fake news relating to coronavirus reporting and other forms of censorship, which, according to organizations like RSF, International Press Institute, and Human Rights Watch, were mere pretences of fighting the spread of the virus (ibid.). These measures indicate the dearth of trust been government and the media in certain countries, hence the need for control and censorship. In the US, President Trump accused media outlets such as CNN of "doing everything they can to instil fear in the people" (Karni, 2020). Trust in the media by the public and political leadership is essential during a crisis like a pandemic where information about the risk is required to change people's attitudes and behaviours related to COVID-19. Distrust in the media can be detrimental to the pandemic response.

Post-Truth and the Erosion of Trust

The articles *COVID-19: The first post-truth pandemic* (Parmet & Paul, 2020) and *A post-truth pandemic* (Shelton, 2020) aptly capture the political context of public health communication during the pandemic. At the same time as the pandemic was highly data-driven, another phenomenon was unfolding – shifting society towards a "post-truth pandemic" outlook. In 2016, the concept of "post-truth" was named the word of the year by the *Oxford Dictionary*, ostensibly to capture the times characterized by an "obfuscation of facts, abandonment of evidential standards in reasoning" (McIntyre, 2018, p. 1). The *Oxford Dictionary* defines post-truth as "relating to or denoting circumstances in which objective facts are less influential in shaping public opinion than appeals to emotion and personal belief". Post-truth is part of a growing trend where some feel embold-ened to try to bend reality to fit their opinions based on a conviction that facts can always be shaded, selected, and presented within a political context that favours one interpretation of truth over another (McIntyre, 2018, p. 6). Prominent politi-cal leaders in the world have openly misled their people through disinformation and with a brazen disregard for facts and truth. During the Brexit campaign, false statistics were openly advertised on hundreds of buses and politicians openly used disinformation to persuade their polarized camps. The election of Donald Trump as the US president saw an increase in open fact-free communication in the US. For example, on 21 January 2017, the newly appointed White House Press Secretary Sean Spicer accused the media of underestimating the number of people who attended Trump's inauguration ceremony, despite the existence of photographic evidence from many trusted sources. Even though this was a provable falsehood, the White House counsellor to the president defended the claim on the basis that these were "alternative facts". This means that facts are not given and hence there is no single objective truth. The truth is constantly be-ing challenged and disputed.

The era has seen the continued dismantling of the knowledge production sys-tems. Changes in public communications have facilitated the rise of multiple epistemic centres, producing their knowledge, challenging existing knowledge, and vying for public attention, legitimacy, and power. Knowledge production and dissemination have been so decentralized to an extent that the position of experts, journalists and traditional media has been weakened. Knowledge and truth have become fluid. This induces complexity in the epistemic norms of knowledge, belief, acceptance, verification, and perspective. For example, "the collapse of news gatekeeping opens the floodgates to information and misinformation, truth and lies, scientific and unscientific knowledge, facts and fiction" (Waisbord, 2018). All sorts of information flourish in the endless digital spaces, where anti-scientific arguments are produced and disseminated through a complex archi-tecture of communication institutions – think tanks, conferences, legacy media, and social media (Ibid., p. 1871; Mooney, 2007). The labyrinth of information, misinformation and disinformation exacerbates the elusiveness of truth.

In this context, risk and crisis communication messages are no longer grounded on facts only. The media and public leaders alike have peddled lies, misleading and sometimes false information about COVID-19. As Shelton (2020) argues, the most obvious examples of the post-truth pandemic are those "where gov-ernment officials are responsible for obfuscating the reality of the virus and its impact on people, and actively intervening to prevent damaging – but still very much factual – information from being released to the public" (p. 3). Govern-ment officials across the world have deliberately misled the public in pursuit of other competing interests. The barrage of false information has helped erode trust in public health leaders and hinders efforts to contain the pandemic (Parmet & Paul, 2020).

The political context of public health communication is a contested discourse arena where different voices vie to broadly influence policy and decision-making. Many authors contend that truth has become subordinated to politics, with implications for political debates, science, technology, and common sense thinking (de Freitas Araujo, 2022). Not surprisingly, during the pandemic, we witnessed a rise in the partisan-divided trust in scientific facts and statistics on the coronavirus in countries like the USA. Reasons for embracing anti-scientific facts vary across issues, from masks to vaccinations. The emergence of "post-truth" is often associated with the rise of conspiracy theories and the lack of trust in scientific knowledge (Kwok, Singh, & Heimans, 2023). Post-truth inevitably leads to the erosion of trust.

Conclusion

Trust is crucial for the successful containment of a public health crisis. Trust in political leadership, government, public health authorities, the vaccines and the systems that develop and distribute them, the messenger, and the media play an important role in the people's attitudes and behaviours related to COVID-19. Trust impacts the people's willingness to comply with government recommendations and adopt behaviours that reduce the threat of infection. Lack of trust diminishes the possibility of the public adhering to recommendations. Trust is not something that is built during an emergency; it has to be cultivated well before the crisis and mended again after the crisis. Rebuilding trust is crucial for the future management of public health crises. Covello (1992) identifies four factors that are required to build trust: (1) transparency and honesty; (2) empathy and care; (3) dedication and commitment; and (4) competence and expertise.

References

Adamecz-Völgyi, A., & Szabó-Morvai, Á. (2021). Confidence in Public institutions is critical in containing the COVID-19 pandemic. Retrieved from doi:10.2139/ssrn.3867690

Adeitan, M. A., Onyechi, N. J., & Omah, O. (2021). COVID-19 containment and control: Information source credibility and adoption of prevention strategies among residents in South West Nigeria. *Journal of African Media Studies, 13*(2), 235–251. doi:10.1386/jams_00046_1

Afrobarometer. (2022). Angolans trust religious and traditional leaders more than elected leaders, Afrobarometer survey shows. https://www.afrobarometer.org/articles/angolans-trust-religious-and-traditional-leaders-more-than-elected-leaders-afrobarometer-survey-shows/

AllAfrica. (2020). Africa: How billions worth of Covid-19 funds were stolen in Africa. Retrieved from Allafrica.com website. https://allafrica.com/stories/202009070230.html

Arriola, L. R., & Grossman, A. N. (2021). Ethnic Marginalization and (non)compliance in public health emergencies. *The Journal of Politics, 83*(3), 807–820. doi:10.1086/710784

Bertsou, E. (2019). Rethinking political distrust. *European Political Science Review, 11*(2), 213–230. doi:10.1017/S1755773919000080

Blair, R. A., Morse, B. S., & Tsai, L. L. (2017). Public health and public trust: Survey evidence from the Ebola virus disease epidemic in Liberia. *Social Science & Medicine, 172*, 89–97. doi:10.1016/j.socscimed.2016.11.016

Boin, A., Hart, P. t., Stern, E., & Sundelius, B. (2005). *The Politics of Crisis Management: Public Leadership under Pressure.* Cambridge: Cambridge University Press.

Boin, A., McConnell, A., & Hart, P. t. (2008). *Governing after Crisis: The Politics of Investigation, Accountability and Learning.* Cambridge: Cambridge University Press.

Bollyky, T. J., Hulland, E. N., Barber, R. M., Collins, J. K., Kiernan, S., Moses, M., . . . Dieleman, J. L. (2022). Pandemic preparedness and COVID-19: an exploratory analysis of infection and fatality rates, and contextual factors associated with preparedness in 177 countries, from Jan 1, 2020, to Sept 30, 2021. *The Lancet, 399*(10334), 1489–1512. doi:10.1016/S0140-6736(22)00172-6

Bratton, M., & Gyimah-Boadi, E. (2016). *Do trustworthy Institutions Matter for Development? Corruption, Trust, and Government Performance in Africa.* Retrieved from Ghana https://www.afrobarometer.org/wp-content/uploads/migrated/files/publications/Dispatches/ab_r6_dispatchno112_trustworthy_institutions_and_development_in_africa.pdf

Chingwete, A. (2016). *AD90: In South Africa, Citizens' Trust in president, Political Institutions Drops Sharply.* Accra: Afrobarometer.

Covello, V. T. (1992). Trust and credibility in risk communication. *Health and Environment Digest, 6*(1), 1–4.

Daniyal, S. (2020). Coronavirus: Why are Indians running away from isolation wards? Retrieved from https://scroll.in/pulse/956280/is-indians-lack-of-trust-in-public-healthcare-hurting-efforts-to-battle-coronavirus

de Freitas Araujo, S. (2020). Truth, half-truth, and post-truth: Lessons from William James. *Journal of Constructivist Psychology, 35*(2), 478–490. doi:10.1080/10720537.2020.1727390

Demeshko, A., Buckley, L., Morphett, K., Adams, J., Meany, R., & Cullerton, K. (2022). Characterising trusted spokespeople in noncommunicable disease prevention: A systematic scoping review. *Preventive Medicine Reports, 29*, 101934. doi:10.1016/j.pmedr.2022.101934

Dhillon, R. S., & Kelly, J. D. (2015). Community trust and the Ebola endgame. *New England Journal of Medicine, 373*(9), 787–789. doi:10.1056/NEJMp1508413

Ezeibe, C. C., Ilo, C., Ezeibe, E. N., Oguonu, C. N., Nwankwo, N. A., Ajaero, C. K., & Osadebe, N. (2020). Political distrust and the spread of COVID-19 in Nigeria. *Global Public Health, 15*(12), 1753–1766. doi:10.1080/17441692.2020.1828987

Fletcher, R. (2020). Trust will get worse before it gets better. Retrieved from https://www.digitalnewsreport.org/publications/2020/trust-will-get-worse-gets-better/

Geelani, G., & Gupta, I. (2020). Coronavirus runaways pose risk to society, lead to unnecessary panic. *India Today.* Retrieved from https://www.indiatoday.in/mailtoday/story/coronavirus-runaways-pose-risk-to-society-lead-to-unnecessary-panic-1656684-2020-03-17

Grosser, K. M. (2016). Trust in online journalism. *Digital Journalism, 4*(8), 1036–1057. doi:10.1080/21670811.2015.1127174

Henderson, J., Ward, P. R., Tonkin, E., Meyer, S. B., Pillen, H., McCullum, D., . . . Wilson, A. (2020). Developing and maintaining public trust during and post-COVID-19: Can we apply a model developed for responding to food scares? *8.* Retrieved from https://www.frontiersin.org/article/10.3389/fpubh.2020.00369 doi:10.3389/fpubh.2020.00369

Hetherington, M. J. (2005). *Why Trust Matters: Declining Political Trust and the Demise of American Liberalism.* Princetow, NJ: Princeton University Press.

Holt, E. (2021). Media restrictions have "cost lives". *The Lancet, 397*(10286), 1695–1696. doi:10.1016/S0140-6736(21)01053-9

Hovland, C. I., & Weiss, W. (1951). The Influence of source credibility on communication effectiveness*. *Public Opinion Quarterly, 15*(4), 635–650. doi:10.1086/266350 %J Public Opinion Quarterly.

Kapucu, N., & Van Wart, M. (2008). Making matters worse: An anatomy of leadership failures in managing catastrophic events. *Administration & Society, 40*(7), 711–740. doi:10.1177/0095399708323143

Karni, A. (2020). Trump criticizes media for coverage of coronavirus. *The New York Times.* Retrieved from https://www.nytimes.com/2020/02/28/us/politics/cpac-coronavirus.html

Katenda, L. M. (2022). For religious leaders in Africa, popular trust may present opportunity, challenge in times of crisis. Retrieved from https://www.afrobarometer.org/wp-content/uploads/2022/08/AD536-PAP13-For-Africas-religious-leaders-popular-trust-presents-opportunity-and-challenge-Afrobarometer-31july22.pdf

Krippahl, C. (2020, 10.06.2020). COVID-19 in Africa: The need to improve communication. *Deutsche Welle.* Retrieved from https://www.dw.com/en/covid-19-in-africa-the-need-to-improve-communication/a-53762789

Kwok, H., Singh, P., & Heimans, S. (2021). The regime of 'post-truth': COVID-19 and the politics of knowledge. *Discourse: Studies in the Cultural Politics of Education, 44*(1), 106–120. doi:10.1080/01596306.2021.1965544

Lazarus, J. V., Wyka, K., White, T. M., Picchio, C. A., Gostin, L. O., Larson, H. J., . . . El-Mohandes, A. (2023). A survey of COVID-19 vaccine acceptance across 23 countries in 2022. *Nature Medicine, 29*(2), 366–375. doi:10.1038/s41591-022-02185-4

Mansell, R., Livingstone, S., & Tambini. (2019). *Tackling the Information Crisis: A Policy Framework for Media System Resilience.* Retrieved from London https://www.lse.ac.uk/media-and-communications/assets/documents/research/T3-Report-Tackling-the-Information-Crisis.pdf

Marcinkowski, F., & Starke, C. (2018). Trust in government: What's news media got to do with it? *Studies in Communication Sciences, 18*(1), 87–102. doi:10.24434/j.scoms.2018.01.006

Marien, S., & Hooghe, M. (2011). Does political trust matter? An empirical investigation into the relation between political trust and support for law compliance. *European Journal of Political Research, 50*(2), 267–291. doi:10.1111/j.1475-6765.2010.01930.x

Mayer, R. C., Davis, J. H., & Schoorman, F. D. (1995). An Integrative model of organizational trust. *The Academy of Management Review, 20*(3), 709–734. doi:10.2307/258792

McIntyre, L. (2018). *Post-Truth.* Cambridge: MIT Press.

McLean, H., & Ewart, J. (2020). *Political Leadership in Disaster and Crisis Communication and Management. International Perspectives and Practices*. Cham, Switzerland: Palgrave Macmillan.

Miller, A. H. (1974). Political issues and trust in government: 1964–1970. *The American Political Science Review, 68*(3), 951–972. doi:10.2307/1959140

Mooney, C. (2007). *The Republican War on Science*. New York: Basic Books.

Moosa, M., & Hofmeyr, J. (2021). AD474: South Africans' trust in institutions and representatives reaches new low. Retrieved from https://www.afrobarometer.org/wp-content/uploads/2022/02/ad474-south_africans_trust_in_institutions_reaches_new_low-afrobarometer-20aug21.pdf

Moyo, J. (2021) Africa: COVID-19 targets politicians in droves. Anadolu Agency Corporation, Turkey (AA), Retrieved from https://www.aa.com.tr/en/africa/africa-covid-19-targets-politicians-in-droves/2124194# (Accessed 22.06.2023).

Newman, N., Fletcher, R., Robertson, C., Eddy, K., & Nielsen, R. K. (2022). *Digital News Report 2022*. Retrieved from Oxford, UK https://reutersinstitute.politics.ox.ac.uk/sites/default/files/2022-06/Digital_News-Report_2022.pdf

O'Keefe, D. J. (2002). *Persuasion: Theory and Research* (2nd ed.). Thousand Oaks, CA: Sage.

OECD. (2021a). *Building Trust to Reinforce Democracy: Key Findings from the 2021 OECD Survey on Drivers of Trust in Public Institutions*. Paris: OECD.

OECD. (2021b). *Drivers of Trust in Public Institutions in Finland*. Paris: OECD.

OECD. (2021c). *Enhancing Public Trust in COVID-19 Vaccination: The Role of Governments*. Paris: OECD.

OECD. (2022). *Drivers of Trust in Public Institutions in Norway*. Paris: OECD.

OECD. (2023). *Drivers of Trust in Public Institutions in New Zealand*. Paris: OECD.

Parmet, W. E., & Paul, J. (2020). COVID-19: The first posttruth pandemic. *American Journal of Public Health, 110*(7), 945–946. doi:10.2105/AJPH.2020.305721

Pollard, M. S., & Davis, L. M. (2021). *Decline in Trust in the Centers for Disease Control and Prevention during the COVID-19 Pandemic*. Santa Monica, CA: RAND Corporation.

Reporters Without Borders. (2021). 2021 World Press Freedom Index: Journalism, the vaccine against disinformation, blocked in more than 130 countries. Retrieved from https://rsf.org/en/2021-world-press-freedom-index-journalism-vaccine-against-disinformation-blocked-more-130-countries

Richardson, E. T., McGinnis, T., & Frankfurter, R. (2019). Ebola and the narrative of mistrust. *BMJ Global Health, 4*(6), e001932. doi:10.1136/bmjgh-2019-001932

Richardson, S., & Spiegelhalter, D. (2020). Coronavirus statistics: What can we trust and what should we ignore? *The Guardian*. Retrieved from https://www.theguardian.com/world/2020/apr/12/coronavirus-statistics-what-can-we-trust-and-what-should-we-ignore

Seydou, A. (2021). Africa is starting to receive covid-19 vaccines. But do citizens trust their governments to ensure they're safe? Retrieved from https://www.afrobarometer.org/articles/africa-starting-receive-covid-19-vaccines-do-citizens-trust-their-governments-ensure-theyre/

Shelton, T. (2020). A post-truth pandemic? *Big Data & Society, 7*(2), 2053951720965612. doi:10.1177/2053951720965612

Sheppard, B. H., & Sherman, D. M. (1998). The grammars of trust: A model and general implications. *The Academy of Management Review, 23*(3), 422–437. doi:10.5465/amr.1998.926619

Shore, D. A. (2003). Communicating in times of uncertainty: The need for trust. *Journal of Health Communication, 8*(suppl), 13–14. doi:10.1080/713851977

Tessema, G. A., Kinfu, Y., Dachew, B. A., Tesema, A. G., Assefa, Y., Alene, K. A., . . . Tesfay, F. H. (2021). The COVID-19 pandemic and healthcare systems in Africa: a scoping review of preparedness, impact and response. *BMJ Global Health, 6*(12), e007179. doi:10.1136/bmjgh-2021-007179 %J BMJ Global Health

Toff, B., Badrinathan, S., Mont'Alverne, C., Arguedas, A. R., Fletcher, R., & Nielsen, R. K. (2021). *Overcoming Indifference: What Attitudes Towards News Tell Us about Building Trust*. Retrieved from Oxford https://reutersinstitute.politics.ox.ac.uk/sites/default/files/2021-09/Toff%20et%20al%20-%20Overcoming%20Indifference%20FINAL.pdf

Tormala, Z. L., & Clarkson, J. J. (2008). Source trustworthiness and information processing in multiple message situations: A contextual analysis. *Social Cognition, 26*(3), 357–367. doi:10.1521/soco.2008.26.3.357

Van Wart, M. J. P. a. r. (2003). Public-sector leadership theory: An assessment. *Public Administration Review, 63*(2), 214–228.

Waisbord, S. (2018). Truth is what happens to news. *Journalism Studies, 19*(13), 1866–1878. doi:10.1080/1461670X.2018.1492881

Ward, P. R. (2017). Improving access to, use of, and outcomes from public health programs: The importance of building and maintaining trust with patients/clients. *Frontiers in Public Health, 5*(22). doi:10.3389/fpubh.2017.00022

Ward, P. R., Attwell, K., Meyer, S. B., Rokkas, P., & Leask, J. (2017). Understanding the perceived logic of care by vaccine-hesitant and vaccine-refusing parents: A qualitative study in Australia. *PLOS ONE, 12*(10), e0185955. doi:10.1371/journal.pone.0185955

WHO. (2017). WHO strategic communications framework for effective communications. Retrieved from https://www.who.int/mediacentre/communication-framework.pdf

Zmerli, S. (2014). Political Trust. In A. C. Michalos (Ed.), *Encyclopedia of Quality of Life and Well-Being Research* (pp. 4887–4889). Dordrecht: Springer Netherlands.

10 The Infodemic Scourge

Introduction

A successful public health response to an outbreak, epidemic or pandemic, depends on the effective dissemination of accurate messages and compliance with the recommendations. The coronavirus pandemic crisis and its related crises fuelled an unprecedented demand for information and a desire to communicate. Naturally, when a public health crisis unfolds people search for information and knowledge about the risk they face. They turn to all available sources for information, be it digital sources or human sources. In the era of digital communications and social media, sources of information are in overabundance. Information and information-sharing is just a tweet away from the audience, and messages of all sorts travel faster than even the virus itself. In this maze of communication, finding reliable and credible sources is daunting for the audience. Fear, anxiety, curiosity, and uncertainty (both scientific and epistemic) drive conversations offline, in the media and in social media spaces. With the pandemic threat unfolding in a context characterized by diverse digital media ecologies and instantaneous communications, many voices – official or unofficial sources, experts, pundits, denialists, sceptics, and epistemic and counter-epistemic centres – vied for public attention in the communication arena. Consequently, public health messages were muffled by a huge amount of information, including false information, misinformation, disinformation, deceptive information, false rumours, fake news, and conspiracy theories. In contexts where public authorities and the mainstream media lack public trust or are weak, crucial information drown and "polluted messages" become mainstream. In this public communication chaos, in the words of Albert Camus "everything is true, and nothing is true" or in the words of Russian novelist Peter Pomerantsev "nothing is true and everything is possible". This chapter examines the different information disorders that came to the fore during the pandemic. It examines the scourge of misinformation and disinformation, identified by the World Health Organization (WHO) as another disease, "infodemic", and its impact on individual decision-making and the measures to counter it. This chapter also discusses the implications of filter

DOI: 10.4324/9781003401827-10

bubbles and echo chambers on public health communication. It argues that these variants of information disorders obscure health crisis communication messages and consequently undermine crisis containment.

Data-Driven Pandemic

Digital communications and social media have fundamentally changed the way public health information is produced, distributed, and consumed. Developments in cheaper information and communication technologies such as mobile telephones, personal computers, and tablets mean that most people, even more than before, have access to technologies imbued with content production (text, video-editing) and publishing tools. Anyone can produce and disseminate content. Social media, which is driven by user-generated context, provides unlimited spaces for the distribution and consumption of such content. Another facet of social media is that the consumption of information, which in the past was purely a private affair, has now become public. When social media users consume content on their platforms, they react to that content by liking, commenting, and sharing it with other users in their networks. Any interactions the user does with the information trigger other inbuilt algorithm settings that also ensure that popular content is seen and shared even wider with other social media users. The speed with which information travels in social media means that "popular" information spreads like wildfire in dry grass. The pace of information dissemination is supercharged. Gone are the days when people will wait for news updates on their television and news stations. While traditional media works within the confines of journalism – in seeking, verifying, and publishing news – ordinary citizens with a story to share can do so at a fraction of what it used to cost. This information can be passed unfiltered and in real time between "friends" in the vast social media network. Social recommendations drive readership in social media as people rely on stories liked or shared by friends in their network. Social media enables instantaneous dissemination and retribution of information.

The amount of data generated, analysed, and consumed about the coronavirus led some to proclaim that this is the first "data-driven pandemic" (Shelton, 2020). However, high-speed digital communication creates an overabundance of information, both scientific and anti-scientific. The pervasiveness of social media misinformation makes it difficult for the public to discern what is true and what is false. This has had negative repercussions on the public responses to the coronavirus pandemic. Most worrying is the predominance of bots in social media discussions. In one study, researchers found that bots may account for between 45% and 60% of Twitter accounts discussing COVID-19 and that many of these have been spreading and amplifying misinformation and conspiracy theories (Hao, 2020). The global nature of both the pandemic and social media explains the surge of messages from a large swath of actors motivated by different interests. Communication technologies make it easier for these actors to disseminate their messages widely.

COVID-19 Information Disorders

Variants of "information disorders" (Wardle & Derakhshan, 2017) predates the COVID-19 pandemic. A cursory look at history reveals that misinformation and disinformation are not new phenomena. The recent interest in the subject stems from the surge in the spread of misinformation on digital communication channels such as social media, where gatekeeping or news filtering powers have been eroded. Manipulated and fabricated information, clickbait headlines, imposter content, fake news, memes, satire, and parody pollute social media networks and in some cases, enter the mainstream media, thus compounding the COVID-19 messages. Social media and other digital platforms fuelled increases in these information disorders at a pace we have not witnessed during previous epidemics and pandemics. The coronavirus pandemic ushered in exponential growth in the flow of information, both correct and incorrect, about the COVID-19 pandemic. Not surprisingly, WHO identified "infodemic" and "disinfodemic" as another disease accompanying the COVID-19 pandemic. The WHO uses the notion of "infodemic" to refer to "an overabundance of information – some accurate and some not – that makes it hard for people to find trustworthy sources and reliable guidance when they need it". Finding credible information on social media is like looking for a needle in a haystack. "Disinfodemic" refers to the spread of misinformation and disinformation.

Several concepts have been used to capture variants of information disorder. There is however a lack of absolute clarity in the conceptualisations, and hence no clear delineations between the concepts. Boundaries between accurate information and misinformation are fluid, and this presents a constant challenge to researchers across fields. In their article "Information Disorder: Toward an Interdisciplinary Framework for Research and Policy Making", Wardle and Derakhshan (2017) identify three different types: misinformation, disinformation, and malinformation. These types are further categorized between two dimensions: false and harmful. Misinformation is when false information is shared, but *no harm is meant*; disinformation is when false information is knowingly shared *to cause harm*; and malinformation is when genuine information is shared *to cause harm*, often by moving information designed to stay private into the public sphere. Malinformation refers to information that is based on reality but is used to inflict harm on a person, organisation, or country. Wardle and Derakhshan (2018, p. 44) further clarify the differences between the two notions of misinformation and disinformation:

1 Misinformation is information that is false, but the person who is disseminating it believes that it is true.
2 Disinformation is information that is false, and the person who is disseminating it knows it is false. It is a deliberate, intentional lie.

Misinformation and disinformation are distinguished by the degree of the intent behind the false information shared (Kligler-Vilenchik, 2021).

Wardle and Derakhshan (2018) describe three types of information disorders and the various guises of false and potentially harmful information. They further distinguish the elements in the information disorder, that is, the agent, the message, and the interpreters. They also emphasized the creation, production, and distribution phases. Important is the understanding of the identity and motives of the agents who create fabricated messages, those who produce the messages, those who distribute the message, and finally those who consume them. Information pollution involves many actors, including the mainstream media, which has amplified some of the disinformation. For instance, the mainstream media were accused of amplifying some of former US President Trump's tweets, some of which peddled false or conspiracy narratives. The information disorder, which takes various forms, may be spread fast through various communication channels. The framework by Wardle and Derakhshan (2018) emphasizes distinguishing messages that are true from those that are false, and also those that are true (and those messages with some truth) but which are created, produced, or distributed by "agents" who intend to harm rather than serve the public interests (ibid., p. 44). However, in the so-called post-truth era, truth is no longer a taken-for-granted phenomenon.

Fake News in Pandemic Times

The coronavirus pandemic witnessed a huge increase in the dissemination of fake news. Fake news is a controversial concept that has been used in different contexts. Even though the concept had been used before to refer to news that was not true, former US President Donald Trump took the concept to the mainstream during his election campaign in 2016. As noted in the BBC, President Trump took the phrase "fake news" and co-opted it to mean news he simply didn't like or news that he didn't want his supporters to hear, and this news was further labelled as the enemy of the people (D. Lee, 2018). Other political leaders in other parts of the world, including Bolsonaro in Brazil, Duterte in the Philippines, and politicians in the UK and Australia, used the concept as shorthand to say "don't believe that, trust me" (ibid.). As such, the concept has been used as a political tool to discredit the mainstream media. Not surprisingly, at the onset of the pandemic, trust in mainstream media was at its lowest, especially in the US. In academic circles, fake news has been defined as "news articles that are intentionally and verifiably false and could mislead readers" (Allcott & Gentzkow, 2017, p. 213). This information can be difficult to spot, as it comes under many guises.

Fake news appears in many different forms, which explains why it is sometimes difficult to identify it. Wardle (2017) identifies seven categories of fake news:

- *False connection* (where headlines, visuals, or captions do not support the content)
- *False context* (when genuine content is shared with false contextual information)

- *Manipulated context* (when genuine information or imagery is manipulated to deceive)
- *Fabricated content* (news content is 100% false, designed to deceive and do harm)
- *Imposter content* (when genuine sources are impersonated)
- *Misleading content* (misleading use of information to frame an issue or individual)
- *Satire or parody* (no intention to cause harm but has the potential to fool)

From this overview, fake news can either be wholly false or contain deliberately misleading elements incorporated within its content or context (Bakir & McStay, 2018). It is misleading because it is a production that resembles real news articles that are associated with the works of professional journalists, who are expected to provide reliable, accurate, and comprehensive information. Real news often goes through editorial processes that save as gatekeepers and ensure adherence to journalistic principles. The digitalisation of media has made it easy to create news articles and also different forms of fake news such as "serious fabrications, large-scale hoaxes and humorous fakes" (Rubin, Chen, & Conroy, 2015). Fake news articles have impersonated well-known news sources like CNN and BBC.

Fake news can be found in both old and new media. There are many motivations behind the production and dissemination of fake news. Tandoc et al. (2018) identify two main motives behind fake news: financial and ideological. Content providers motivated by financial gains produce news articles that are most likely to attract viewers, especially in the social media arena. They rely on the exploits of social media and other digital communication platforms where views and shares are converted into advertising revenues. They use eye-catching clickbait such as headlines, visuals, and pictures to gain the attention and curiosity of the users. They entice the users to click on items, follow links, and read, all with the main aim of increasing traffic and profit. Yellow press, tabloids, and online news outlets present to their readers a spectrum of unverified news through eye-catching headlines, exaggerations, or sensationalism. Large-scale hoaxes attempt to deceive audiences by masquerading as news; these can easily be mistakenly validated in mainstream news sources.

During the pandemic, we witnessed several forms of fake news, distributed mainly on social media platforms such as Facebook and Twitter, but also in some media outlets. In "Analysis of fake news disseminated during the COVID-19 pandemic in Brazil", Barcelos (2020) found that most fake news was spread through WhatsApp and Facebook and that the most frequent thematic categories were politics, epidemiology, statistics (proportion of cases and deaths), and prevention. Misinformation about the number of cases and deaths and prevention measures and treatment were registered around the world. Fake news stories continue to fool and mislead millions of readers around the world. A poll by Ofcom in the UK found that almost half (46% of the UK population) had been exposed to fake news about the coronavirus and 40% were finding it hard to know what was true or false about the virus (Ofcom, 2020).

Fake news has a huge implication on public health communication messages during a pandemic. In a crisis like a pandemic, where human life is at stake, access to accurate, trustworthy, and credible sources of information can save lives. Fake news, just like other information disorders, can undermine the effectiveness of the messages. Fake news keeps citizens wrongly informed, and wrong information is likely to mislead citizens into distrusting and rejecting correct and useful information from authorities. In some cases, fake news may lead people to be emotionally antagonized against political decisions. Wrong information can affect the way individuals understand the risks associated with the virus. Wrong information about a virus may give people wrong advice about what to do and how best to manage their health and well-being. It can also lead people to make wrong decisions and cause unnecessary panic and confusion. It affects people's attitude towards the virus, other people, and public authorities. It generates confusion in society and undermines the effectiveness of pandemic management. Another dimension of fake news is that it adds to the information flood and may lead to the drowning of crucial information.

Beliefs in Conspiracy Theories

The COVID-19 pandemic became a fertile ground for all sorts of conspiracy theories, with negative ramifications on public health messages. As Knight notes:

> The coronavirus pandemic is a perfect storm for conspiracy theories. Some people have had a lot of time on their hands, and little social contact. Social media mean misinformation can spread quickly and widely. Conspiracy theories have flourished.
>
> (Peter Knight[1])

The *Merriam-Webster* dictionary defines a conspiracy theory as "a theory that explains an event or set of circumstances as the result of a secret plot by usually powerful conspirators". Conspiracy and secrecy are hence intractably linked. Conspiracy theory is the belief that nothing happens by accident, nothing is as it seems, and everything is connected (Barkun, 2013). There is a wide range of conspiracy theories and Barkun (2013) divides these into three broad categories: *event conspiracies, systemic conspiracies*, and *super conspiracies*. Event conspiracies constellate around specific single events. Notable examples are conspiracies that underpin the 11 September 2001 terrorist attacks on the USA, the assassination of JFK Kennedy, and the spread of AIDS in the black communities. In systemic conspiracies, the goals of the conspirators are broad and sweeping (e.g. trying to gain control over a country or region). In super conspiracies, multiple conspiracies converge.

Conspiracy theories are often supported with an elaborate presentation of "evidence" to substantiate the claims. Where proof is difficult to ascertain, the theorist claim that conspiracists, due to their power, control the means of knowledge production and dissemination to mislead those that seek to expose them. Belief in a conspiracy theory is a matter of faith rather than proof (Barkun, 2013). A conspiracy theory is a shared belief system providing an alternative ideological framework to explain a situation (Leonard & Philippe, 2021). Because it is a belief, a conspiracy theory is very difficult to contain.

Conspiracy theories of various natures are prevalent. More important for this work are those conspiracy theories that impact on public health communication, that is, conspiracy theories that undermine or create distrust towards public health messages. Conspiracy theories build on the distrust of the "other". The spread of conspiracy theories during public health crises is exacerbated by mistrust towards the mainstream media, the public authorities, and government institutions. Public health crises and diseases often attract speculation and rumours. In his book *An Epidemic of Rumours: How stories shape our perception of disease*, Jon De Lee notes that "societies usually respond to the eruption of disease by constructing stories, jokes, conspiracy theories, legends, and rumours, but these narratives are often more damaging than the disease they reference" (J. D. Lee, 2014). Diseases such as the 2003 SARS epidemic, AIDS, H1N1, avian flu, Ebola, and of late, COVID-19 have comparative conspiracy theory narratives. Likewise, COVID-19 conspiracy theories have proliferated during the pandemic. What is peculiar about the COVID-19 conspiracy theories is their amplification in social media, which has expanded their reach into society. This means that COVID-19 conspiracy theories are easily accessible across the world.

Some conspiracy theories focus on the origins, spread, and cure of the disease. Since the virus was first detected in the Chinese city of Wuhan, it is still a mystery how the virus emerged. The question of how the virus emerged has been pursued in the digital environment. Today, there are many strands of narratives seeking to answer the question of how the virus emerged. One of the dominant COVID-19 narratives is that the virus originated in a meat market in Wuhan through human contact with an infected animal. Even though it was a common-sense justification of using the place of origin as an identifier, it is problematic, in that it links the infection with an ethnicity. As Humphreys (2002) argues in "No Safe Place: Disease and Panic in American History", identifying the virus by its source leads to the racialisation of the disease. It is precisely for these reasons that the WHO does not use geographical names as disease identifiers; hence the use of the Delta COVID-19 variant instead of the Indian variant and the Alpha variant instead of the Kent variant. Former US President Donald Trump repeatedly referred to the coronavirus as the "Chinese virus" and announced the suspension of travel from Europe to protect Americans from the foreign virus. The racialized language led to a surge of racist acts and harassment of the Asian

American community in the USA. The Department of Homeland Security even issued a warning that white supremacists may exploit the crisis against Asian Americans.

Closely linked to the Chinese origins of the virus is another narrative that the coronavirus originated from a laboratory in Wuhan, China. Some strands of the narrative hold that the virus was accidentally leaked from a Chinese laboratory. This theory is mainstream, given the insinuations by US leaders. So strong is the theory that President Biden even ordered the US intelligence agencies to investigate the origin of the virus, and one of the hypotheses being looked at was that the pandemic originated from a Chinese lab. However, some have previously suggested that COVID-19 came from a US laboratory instead and was potentially brought to China by the US military delegation that was participating in the Military World Games in Wuhan in October 2019. Given the strained relations between China and the US, some give credence to the lab theory, more particularly to the likelihood of a bioweapons race. In this theory, "China's proliferation of bioweapons presents an external danger in the form of security threat from a potentially hostile political rival" (Hartman et al., 2021, p. 4). The more scientific uncertainty surrounds the origins of the disease, the more traction it gains in the narratives.

The lab narratives on viruses revolve around notions of man-made bioweapons unleashed towards certain ethnicities, countries, and even age groups (J. D. Lee, 2014) or accidental release of the virus. In her book *Once Upon a Virus: AIDS legends and Vernacular Risk Perception*, Diane Goldstein recounts three main stories concerning the origins of AIDS, and one of them is that "AIDS is a man-made virus manufactured either accidentally or deliberately in a laboratory (Goldstein, 2004, p. 80). There are also narratives that AIDS originated from US biological testing (Treichler, 1999) and a widely held belief by the African Americans that the CIA created AIDS as a bioweapon created for the "purposeful destruction" of black people or "an out-of-control germ warfare virus". The infamous experiment on African Americans in the 1932–1972 Tuskegee Syphilis Study, "in which 400 African American men who had syphilis were studied to follow the natural course of the disease, without being even given any information about it nor any treatment even after antibiotics became available", has been used as evidence to support the story (J. D. Lee, 2014, p. 60). Experiments like these boost conspiracy theories and "past conspiracies that were revealed as true have served to fuel the current unjustified conspiracy theories circulating" (Leonard & Philippe, 2021).

Another line of thought links COVID-19 to the 5G mobile networks. There are various forms of narratives built around suspicions about the introduction of the 5G mobile technology. Some claim that the virus is real and is caused and spread by the 5G networks and therefore disrupting the network is necessary to stop the spread of the virus. Believers of this line of thought, the so-called anti-5G movement, have even disrupted 5G stations in the UK, Australia, the USA, and other parts of Europe. In the UK alone, more than 87 arson attacks on 5G installations were registered, and engineers have been verbally abused or physically attacked by members of the public who believe in the 5G conspiracy theories. In one weekend alone, over 50 cell towers, including those that did not then support 5G, in the UK were vandalized (Smith).[2] This conspiracy theory has spread globally via social media networks, despite there being no scientific proof of the claims. UNICEF (Montenegro) noted that almost one-third of the citizens of Montenegro (31%) believe that 5G technology causes and spreads coronavirus and that this is being kept secret so that the companies dealing with this technology can continue to make a significant profit (UNICEF, 2021). Another narrative around the 5G conspiracy is that there is no corona, it is just a hoax, or "a pretence to cover-up to the negative health effects of 5G radiation established by those profiteering from the technology" (Hartman et al., 2021). Seeing COVID-19 as a hoax has repercussions on the risk perception and hence can be detrimental to public health messages.

Some conspiracy theories have targeted influential persons such as Microsoft co-founder Bill Gates and Chief Medical Advisor to the President (USA) Anthony Fauci. Myriad conspiracies target Bill Gates and Fauci, from the origins of the virus to the vaccinations, due to their involvement with global public health, scientific research, big tech companies (especially Gates), and other powerful connections. Even though Gates, through the Bill and Melinda Gates Foundation, committed at least $1.75 billion to the global pandemic response, conspirators still claim that he planned and engineered the coronavirus. Gates Foundation's pandemic preparedness simulations are presented as being part of the plan to unleash the virus. The narratives proceed that the motives behind are to make more money and connive with Fauci and big pharma companies. So elaborate are the conspiracy theories that one finds several small publications in Amazon on the theme. Advancing this theory, Robert F Kennedy jr. (2022) in "*The Real Anthony Fauci: Bill Gates, Big Pharma, and the Global War on Democracy and Public Health (Children's Health Defense)* claims that the "Pharma-funded mainstream media has convinced millions of Americans that Dr Anthony Fauci is a hero. He is anything but". The author narrates that Fauci launched his career during the AIDS crisis by partnering with pharmaceutical companies to sabotage the safe and effective treatment of AIDS. He further accounts:

how Fauci, Gates, and their cohorts use their control of media outlets, scientific journals, key government and quasi-governmental agencies, global intelligence agencies, and influential scientists and physicians to flood the public with fearful propaganda about COVID-19 virulence and pathogenesis and to muzzle debate and ruthlessly censor dissent.

There are claims that Fauci and Gates created the pandemic to make money or control people or that Gates wants to implant monitoring microchips in billions of people through a COVID-19 vaccine. Some claims hold that Bill and Melinda Gates Foundation tested vaccines on children in Africa and India. Others accused Gates of using vaccines for mass depopulation. This line finds traction in certain parts of the world where it converges with Western conspiracies to depopulate other parts of the non-Western world. Gates has previously spoken about the benefits of slowing the rate of population growth in a TED Talk in 2010, and this has been used to boost the theories that he wants to depopulate the world. In one such claim, Gates wants "to eliminate at least 3 billion people in the world, starting in Africa, in a plot involving vaccines" (Swenson, 2021).

A 2019 video featuring Robert Young, a US naturopathic practitioner containing this false claim about Gates, was widely circulated in social media anew just when vaccines became available. An article in *The International Centre for Investigative Reporting*[3] shows that the video was trending online at the same time when African countries were acquiring vaccines for their populations. A link to the video was even attached to a false Twitter account for a popular South African opposition leader, Julius Malema. This claim blends into other narratives where mandatory vaccination is seen as part of the conspiracy to eliminate Africans. Some of the posts claim that Gates "added a sterilization formula to every single vaccine for the last 10 years". The narrative is clearly aimed at inducing fear among the targeted population.

Research shows that there are links between beliefs in conspiracy theories and public reactions to the COVID-19 crisis, for example, increased non-compliance with COVID-19 restriction measures, refusal to take vaccinations, and scepticism towards public authorities. Conspiracy theories have negatively affected vaccine attitudes. Interviews with informants in South Africa, Kenya, and Eswatini shed light on the prevalence of conspiracy theories and how these affect people's perceptions of disease and containment measures. In a focus group discussion held in Nairobi, Kenya, in 2021, comments by discussants indicate the gravity of conspiracy theories:

No, I didn't wear a mask because there was this conspiracy theory that talked of Corona not being an African disease. So, I didn't fear the disease because I believed it's a white people problem. When the news came to Africa, it started looking like politics. Even to date, I have never been mask conscious. I only wear it when I go to a place that requires me to wear one for instance getting into a matatu (taxi) or entering a supermarket. But I have never worn it because of fear of getting infected.

Yes, Corona is real and I know that but I bought into the conspiracy theory of believing that it does not get to Africans. But it later came.

The Challenges of Filter Bubbles and Echo Chambers

Information disorders, such as conspiracy theories, find meaning and amplification in social media. Research shows that social media facilitates the creation of echo chambers. For Nguyen (2020), an echo chamber is an epistemic community. He identifies two distinct social epistemic phenomena, that is, an *epistemic bubble* and an *echo chamber*. An epistemic bubble is "a social epistemic structure in which other relevant voices have been left out, perhaps accidentally", while an echo chamber is " a social epistemic structure from which other relevant voices have been actively excluded and discredited" (Nguyen, 2020). The phenomenon of filter bubbles arises through ordinary processes of social selection and community formation. People tend to gather around friends, family, and those that share their views and interest, and hence are exposed to "narrowed and self-reinforcing epistemic filters, which leaves out contrary views" (ibid.). In echo chambers, insiders are convinced to distrust outsiders. When people endorse certain positions on the coronavirus pandemic or conspiracy theories, they create echo chambers. When one adheres to a narrative, they then seek the presence of like-minded individuals, forming a network (Leonard & Philippe, 2021). The echo chamber spreads the reinforcement of both individual and collective actions and propels the action of disobedience against the public authorities (see Leonard & Philippe, 2021, p. 2). Some examples of this phenomenon are climate change deniers and anti-vaxxers. As Santos (2021) notes, these groups work as structures of epistemic exclusion in which members are isolated or isolate themselves from outside epistemic sources (pp. 109-119). The echo chambers act as a mechanism to reinforce existing opinions and certain beliefs within the group. Members leaning towards certain views about the pandemic get reinforcement and support in their networks. Functionalities in social media platforms like Facebook and Twitter foster misinformation in these echo chambers through their algorithm-based news feed algorithms. Feed algorithms limit the range of information by offering suggested content based on previous searches or consumption. They suggest content like that of the users have already been exposed to. Social media creates "environments in which the opinion, political leaning, or beliefs of users about a topic gets reinforced due to repeated interactions with peers or sources having similar tendencies and attitudes" (Cinelli, De Francisci Morales, Galeazzi, Quattrociocchi, & Starnini, 2021). The challenges of echo chambers and filter bubbles were eminent during the pandemic.

Harmful Assertions

Misleading (False) Remedies

The scourge of infodemic has been more visible during the coronavirus pandemic than any other pandemics or epidemics before; much of this can be attributed to virtually anyone with a smart telephone who can easily share with their audiences worldwide grim pictures of the sick and the dead. The fear of the coronavirus, coupled with the absence of approved medicine to treat COVID-19, has been a key driving factor behind the spread of infodemic and disinfodemic. The spread of misleading medical advice claims and false information has been circulated widely on media and social media and some with fatal consequences. Some of the remedies were attributed to scientists, doctors, and other well-known personalities. Social media users across the world have at one point received or even shared a message that purports a remedy for the treatment or management of COVID-19. Why do people share messages on remedies for COVID-19? First, the urge to share such information is driven by a conscious desire to save the lives of friends and those in one's network. They share the message because they believe in it and hope that by sharing, they are helping others to find a remedy for a serious illness. Second, sometimes sharing is purely based on malice to deliberately mislead the public. Third, some people share messages because they are motivated by opportunity of marketing. A good example is the marketing of traditional Asian medicine.

Traditional Asian Medicine

Asian countries have a long history of traditional medicine developed through observation and experience accumulated over thousands of years. Traditional Chinese Medicine (TCM) is one of the oldest forms of medicine in the world. During the outbreak, China used the opportunity to promote the use of TCM as a way to treat the disease.[4] A White Paper, "Fighting COVID-19 China in Action" (2020),[5] highlights the administration of TCM and Western drugs in the treatment of COVID-19 patients. On TCM, the report states that "China has leveraged the unique strength of TCM in pre-emptive prevention, differentiated medication, and multi-targeted intervention, and at every step of COVID-19 treatment and control", and "TCM hospitals were used in the treatment of COVID-19 patients", and claims that "TCM drugs and herbal formulas have proved effective in treating different types of COVID-19 patients". Some of these remedies have been published in prominent English news outlets like *China Daily*, where they reach international readers. In an article, "6 effective TCM recipes for COVID-19" (24.03.2020), the *China Daily* provides a list of TCM medicines that "have proved to be effective in treating the infection".[6] Such claims from Chinese authorities evoke fierce debates in many forums due to the lack of scientific documentation to back the claims. Contestations over the effectiveness of TCM provide a fertile ground for debates, with some promoting and recommending TCM as a remedy for COVID-19 and others denouncing the claims as simple propaganda.

Social media provides a convenient place for spreading information on remedies. On 12 June 2020, Health Analytics Asia published an article, "100 fake COVID-19 WhatsApp forwards that we almost believed".[7] It collated false claims circulated in WhatsApp, a popular social media platform in Asia and other parts of the world. In this article, a team of doctors and fact-checkers collected and debunked widely circulated messages related to COVID-19 remedies. One of the WhatsApp messages claim that the coronavirus remains in the throat for four days before reaching the lungs. This is the time when the person starts coughing or having pain in the throat. Drinking a mixture of warm water and salt or vinegar will kill the virus. Another message suggests that the use of *rasam*, a soup-like concoction of herbs, tamarind juice, and lentils is the best way to cure the coronavirus. Another popular claim is that COVID-19 virus can be killed at a temperature of 30–35 degrees, hence drinking hot water and exposure to the sun for a long time is an effective remedy. The message advices people not to drink ice. Another claim is that the pH value of the novel coronavirus ranges between 5.5 and 8.5, and therefore, one should consume alkaline food that is above the pH level of the virus so as to prevent its spread. This recommendation is attributed to research published in the *Journal of Virology*. The message further lists the pH values of different food items such as lemon, orange, garlic, and avocado, among others. Another message claims that the Chinese are not taking any medicine or any vaccine for coronavirus. Every house has a coronavirus case. They have stopped going to the hospital for a cure. They instead kill the virus by using hot steam inhalation from a kettle four times a day. They do hot gargles and take hot tea four times a day. It claims that the virus is eliminated on the fourth day. Other remedies include the use of ginger, cutting onions into small pieces and eating without water, breathing hot air from a sauna or hairdryer, and using Betadine Sore Throat Gargle to eliminate or minimize the germs while they are still in the throat (before dripping down to the lungs). A remedy attributed to a professor at Beijing Military Hospital claims that slices of lemon in a cup of lukewarm water can save your life. Other users share a remedy proven by an old Chinese doctor that the virus can be cured using boiled garlic water. Another claim, attributed to the WHO, says that no vegetarian has been affected by coronavirus because it requires animal fat in the body to survive.

Many messages on remedies were attributed to well-known personalities and eminent doctors. One such viral message suggesting 22 steps to protect from a coronavirus infection is attributed to renowned Indian cardiac surgeon Dr Devi Shetty. A long post written in Bengali points out 22 suggestions by Dr Shetty, the chairman and founder of Narayana Health. From the sample of messages debunked by Health Analytics Asia, one notes the transnationality of the remedy claims. While it is tempting to regard some remedies as false and as misinformation, people around the world have natural remedies for illnesses like colds, coughs, and the flu. Examples such as passion fruit and onion tea (The Dominican Republic), ginger tea (Cambodia), garlic tea (Mexico), cinnamon tea (Mexico), lemon leaves (Mali), and herbal steam (Zambia) are some known folk remedies. TCM has seen a surge in popularity across the world. When people across the world face a similar threat, they share remedies in abundance on social media. Messages on herbal cures travel fast through social media networks promising cheaper solutions to fight the coronavirus.

Africa: Banking on Herbal Remedies

Much of the infodemic in Africa revolves around the issue of remedies for COVID-19. African countries are characterized by huge inequalities and fragility in health care. Most countries suffer chronic shortages of medicines, medical facilities, and staff. Unlike in the West, where the countries feared that the health sector will be overwhelmed and collapse, the stark reality is that in most parts of Africa, modern health care is limited or even non-existent. People are left on their own to find alternative medical remedies. Traditional medicines have been part of life in Africa, as in other parts of the world, since time immemorial and many still believe in the power of traditional herbs. Traditional medicine has been passed from generation to generation and constitutes a significant part of the African heritage. As UN Educational, Scientific, and Cultural Organization (UNESCO, 2020) correctly notes, in Africa, traditional medicine is culturally entrenched, accessible, and affordable, and serves as a primary source of healthcare for more than 80% of the population across the continent. People across Africa embrace traditional remedies, as these are at least within their immediate reach. In times of adversity, some people turn to traditional practices.

In the absence of known modern medicines, social media and even mainstream media have curated messages promoting traditional remedies. The messages discussed in the Asian case have also been widely circulated in Africa. These messages gave credence to traditionalists – herbalists, healers, and the public – on the existence of alternative medicine. Some of these traditional herbs have existed in pre-colonial Africa. In the absence of modern medicine, people are likely to embrace what is available even if it is contrary to the recommendations of public health authorities. Public health communicators in Africa hence found themselves in a quandary. When they campaign for the uptake of conventional medicine (scientifically tested) and are silent on traditional medicine (known but not scientifically tested), they raise epistemological controversies. To some pundits, not acknowledging the effectiveness of traditional herbs is akin to suppressing traditional knowledge. These epistemological challenges provoke debate, and these debates are futile grounds for infodemic and disinfodemic.

One notable controversy has surrounded the touting of Madagascar's herbal cure, Covid-Organics, as a remedy for COVID-19. Extracted from a local plant and introduced in the country by the Malagasy Institute of Applied Research, the herbal remedy generated a lot of news in both the mainstream and social media. The remedy was fronted by the country's President Andry Rajoelina, and this resonated well with other African leaders whose own nations have a long history of relying on traditional medicine. Pictures of the Madagascar president drinking the remedy at a news conference cemented his claim that it was safe. Despite misgivings by the WHO, which gave a statement that the organisation did not recommend "self-medication with any medicines … as a prevention or cure for COVID-19", several countries in Africa received or purchased Covid-19

Organics. These include Tanzania, Equatorial Guinea, the Central African Republic, the Republic of Congo, the Democratic Republic of Congo, Liberia, and Guinea Bissau. Despite the lack of scientific data on COVID-19 Organic and other traditional remedies, some leaders and other prominent figures have actively promoted these remedies in media and social media. One notable figure who actively promoted traditional remedies is the late Tanzania President Magufuli. He urged the public in Tanzania to shun Western media and embrace traditional medicines and went even further by stopping the testing of people for the deadly virus.

Messages by political leaders undermine messages from public health experts and global institutions like the WHO. In a statement issued by the Regional Office for Africa, WHO (2020) reiterates that the organisation supports scientifically proven traditional medicine:

> WHO recognizes that traditional, complementary and alternative medicine has many benefits and Africa has a long history of traditional medicine and practitioners that play an important role in providing care to populations. Medicinal plants such as Artemisia annua are being considered as possible treatments for COVID-19 and should be tested for efficacy and adverse side effects. Africans deserve to use medicines tested to the same standards as people in the rest of the world. Even if therapies are derived from traditional practice and natural, establishing their efficacy and safety through rigorous clinical trials is critical.

The African Ministers of Health adopted a resolution urging all member states to produce evidence on the safety, efficacy, and quality of traditional medicine. Even though these remedies have not been tested, ordinary citizens in Africa are being exposed, mainly through social media, to misinformation and disinformation about the effectiveness of certain remedies against COVID-19. Evidence is not necessary, but trust in traditional remedies influences behaviours on the ground. The following quotation by a Tanzanian captures the role of trust:

> I honestly don't understand why everyone cast doubt on the effectiveness of traditional herbs in treating modern-day diseases like coronavirus. We must trust our indigenous knowledge of things.[8]

As reported in the Voice of America, herbal cures for COVID-19 have been spreading in Tanzania despite a lack of evidence that they work (Kombe, 2020). The government promoted the use of steam therapy, which entails a concoction of local herbs, although health experts say there is no evidence of its effectiveness against the coronavirus. The government also advised people to eat ginger, garlic, watermelon, oranges, and lemons to boost their immunity. Health Minister Dorothy Gwajima called upon citizens to follow the directives given by health experts such as washing hands with soap and use of steaming and traditional medicines to prevent infections.[9] Government communications provided mixed messages, some of which constitute misinformation (misleading information) while some of the information is correct (maintaining a healthy diet). The danger with mixed messages is that it leads to confusion and even builds a false sense of security. Public health communicators warned that claims about traditional remedies give the public a false sense of security and lead to complacency. People who took remedies promoted by the government and other influential figures (including traditional healers) might feel they are protected from COVID-19 and engage in risky behaviour such as not complying with social distancing.

Interviews in Kenya, South Africa, and Eswatini highlight the proliferation of herbal medicine claims in social media.

Excerpts from Interviews in South Africa

- "I bought eucalyptus oil and used it to steam mainly if I had gone out to the shops".
- "For me, I would drink apple cider vinegar as I heard that it kills the virus in the throat before it goes to the lungs. I would also drink lemon water and honey and drink that every day".
- "I did the steaming and also drank 'umhlonyane'" (local herbs).
- "Umhlonyane is one of the muthi's we grew up drinking, our grand-mothers told us to drink especially if you have flu".
- "Its been a cure for flu for centuries for as long as I can remember".
- "That's why I would drink it because I knew if I drink it, I will get better".
- "Used to drink 'Bloekomboom', it's also a herb from a tree. You cut the roots and also boil like mhlonyane" (Blooekomboom is the Afrikaans name for eucalyptus).
- "I would walk to stadium nearby where there are lots of Blooekomboom and get it from there".
- "On a personal experience, I have seen people who combine the eucalyptus and mhlonyane/lengana and steam with it, they actually feel relief in their chest. You know with Covid symptoms they would feel as though there is a truck sitting on their lungs. But after steaming with the two they can breathe. You know the mechanical changes in the lungs and the oil that has a certain effect on the lungs that opens up the lungs. Cos covid seems to be within the lungs".
- "I remember there was now even a shortage of eucalyptus at Dischem (pharmacy) because everyone was just buying it".
- "My family and I drink traditional herbs like pipiribomb and lengana, these help especially if you feel like you are coming down with a cold or cough".

Excerpts from Focus Group Discussions in Kenya

- "I heard about it (ginger, garlic and honey) from people and then I began to Google. I heard that ginger would heal someone and all they had to do was gurgle warm salty water. And I did all these things and now it was out of fear because initially, I didn't believe that Corona was real but now I was experiencing the symptoms and I knew after Googling that I was indeed infected. I would look up people who were in the USA who said they had contracted the disease and read about their experiences. Then now I'd follow what people said about what to take".
- "Correct. Then I had a cousin of mine who would send me instructions on what I needed to do. They said I should exercise so that my lungs could open up because I was panting a lot".

Faith-Themed Misinformation

Religious-themed misinformation has been a cause for concern during the pandemic, as some of the messages undermined scientific-based messages. While the world grappled with the coronavirus pandemic, religious leaders around the world downplayed the virus and even offered prayers as a plausible remedy. An article in *The Guardian* (Wilson, 2020) shows how prominent religious leaders in the US have downplayed the COVID-19 danger, claiming that the virus was either a hoax or can be defeated by faith in God. The remedy for the virus is by spiritual means rather than solid healthcare policy. Prominent Pentecostal pastor Rodney Howard-Browne is one of the religious leaders in the USA who has undermined public health messages in the US, refusing to call off services in compliance with social distancing measures, even insisting that his congregants embrace and shake hands. He was arrested for defying social distancing orders in the state of Florida.[10] In Alabama, Roy Moore told his followers on Facebook to continue church assemblies: "our faith requires it, our duty demands it, and no law or government can prohibit it" (Wilson, 2020). Another prominent pastor, Kenneth Copeland, told viewers on his Victory Channel that the coronavirus was a "weak strain of flu, and fearing the pandemic was a sin" (ibid.) Other religious figures in the USA have been accused of undermining scientific information, perpetuating conspiracy theories, and generally undermining public health information, discrediting the CDC (Centers for Disease Control and Prevention) and the media.

Similar trends have been observed in the Sub-Saharan African context. In their article in *The Conversation*, Kirby et al. (2020) reflect on the spiritualisation of the pandemic in different African settings. They examine the influence of prominent Pentecostal pastors on public health messaging. They note that "many Pentecostal Christians in Africa as well as other continents, portray the coronavirus as a 'spiritual force of evil' rather than as a biomedical disease". Such perceptions imply that remedies to the pandemic are spiritual rather than medical interventions. A prominent pastor in Zimbabwe, Prophet Emmanuel Makandiwa, reassured his congregation that they will be spared from the virus through prayer and divine protection: "you will not die because the Son is involved in what we are doing … the freedom that no medication can offer". The remedies proffered for the virus are spiritual.

In Tanzania, the late President John Magufuli alarmed health experts when he asserted that divine power would offer protection from the virus: "Coronavirus will be defeated by the Holy Spirit, so we don't have to fear it (Muhumuza, 2020). Even though his government was involved in social distancing campaigns, Magufuli declared that churches and mosques would not be closed because it is where God and "true healing" are found. The Tanzanian president even went further to declare three days of national prayer to help defeat the coronavirus (Voice of America, 2020). Social media is awash with videos of Tanzanians responding to the call for prayers. This is a clear case of messages that undermine public health crisis management.

In Uganda, senior pastor Augustine Yiga was arrested and charged with spreading false information in his televised speeches where he told the public that there was no coronavirus in Africa.[11] These messages muddle risk and crisis communication messages and lead to complacency among the followers. In interviews conducted in Eswatini, the religious influences are visible, as shown in the following excerpts:

> The messages [from the government] were not very clear for me since my passion remains with the people and I am of the view that God is protecting us against this COVID 19.
> I had a difficult time complying with the messages because of my faith and calling.
> I felt this was a test from the evil one to make me relax in my spiritual journey and also challenge my faith in God.
> I also think my faith is working for me.
> I have not taken the vaccine up to now because I think there is a lot of evil attached to the vaccine.
>
> (Interviews Eswatini)

Religious reasoning influences public decisions on vaccination. In their article "Religious Exception for Vaccination or Religious excuses for avoiding vaccination", Pelčić et al. (2016) examine religious influences on vaccination. They note that sections of the public reject vaccination based on religion or they give religious excuses for avoiding vaccination. Religious groups such as the Catholics and the Orthodox have raised concerns about the use of cell lines derived from a voluntarily aborted foetus. The Islamic faith forbids the use of certain food. Pig flesh is forbidden (*haram*) while other animals are licit (*halal*) depending on how they die. The problem is reflected in the use of gelatin in medical products. If gelatin is obtained from a halal animal, then it is permissible to use. The law of necessity is observed when there are no alternatives and the goal of the intervention is to preserve life (ibid). Vaccination refusal based on religion is found in most parts of the world. Certain religions prohibit vaccination for their members. Iannelli (2022) notes that churches that rely on faith healing have an absolute rejection to vaccines. In the USA, except for Mississippi and West Virginia, members of these groups are exempt from immunisation on the basis of religious beliefs. Anti-vaccination groups have exploited grey zones in religious interpretations in their quest to avoid immunisation or to discourage others from getting vaccinated. Iannelli (2022) argues that for many religious groups, anti-vaccine views aren't always about religion. Sometimes, the issues are more social and political. Ethical issues are raised concerning the components of the vaccine and the morality question of the practice of vaccination. The link between religion and vaccines provides fertile grounds for misinformation and disinformation, as pundits take to the media and other information outlets to spread their belief in spiritual healing (hence dispelling science). Groups opposed to the vaccines have taken to social media and other digital communication platforms to front their cause using religious frames

Religious communication messages are not always in tandem with those of public health authorities. The messages sometimes, if not often, contradict those of the health authorities. They sometimes undermine scientific evidence by emphasising the prominence of divine intervention. Religion provides a basis for anti-vaccination information campaigns, with influential religious leaders dispelling other scientific facts about the disease or dissuading their followers not to take the vaccination. As Dwoskin (2021) notes in her article in *The Washington Post*, "On social media, vaccine misinformation mixes with extreme faith":

Some churches and Christian ministries with large online followings – as well as Christian influencers on Facebook, Instagram, TikTok, Twitter and YouTube – are making false claims that vaccines contain foetal tissue or microchips or are construing associations between vaccine ingredients and the devil.

Misinformation and conspiracy theories about the use of foetal tissue from aborted children as ingredients in the development of COVID-19 vaccines gained traction in the digital media. As Jenkins (2022) notes, "some of the abortion opponents have refused to get a coronavirus vaccine because of a distant link to foetal tissue in their development". Moderna, Pfizer-BioNtech, and Johnson & Johnson used cell lines in various ways that trace their origins to aborted foetuses from the 1970s and 1980s (ibid.). Vaccine sceptics have exploited these linkages to frame the vaccine otherwise in a manner that put them in conflict with religious beliefs.

Another theory draws on a Biblical allusion to the satanic "mark of the beast", an apocalyptic verse in the Book of Revelation (Revelation 13: 16-18). It links the vaccines theory that the Antichrist will test Christians by asking them to put a mark on their bodies (Dwoskin, 2021). Taking a vaccine was akin to having a microchip implant. Flourishing in social media are claims that COVID-19 has 666 written all over. A video by Lackey in July – "Could vaccines be the mark of the beast" – was viewed over 100,000 times (ibid.). The internet is awash with videos about the "mark of the beast" misinformation on COVID-19 vaccines and mandates. This example is illustrative of the potency of health misinformation and theories targeting religious audiences. This kind of misinformation is difficult to correct when it is collaborated by influential religious opinion leaders. Some religious leaders have perpetuated this misinformation to dissuade their followers from taking vaccines. The infodemic has had huge implications on the acceptance of vaccinations worldwide.

Scientific Misinformation and COVID-19 Vaccines

Besides the religious-themed misinformation, there has been a proliferation of scientific misinformation in social media. In the history of diseases, vaccines have been central to the prevention of infectious diseases. In the last century, highly effective vaccines have been developed to combat several diseases leading to a growing number of vaccine-preventable diseases. Infectious diseases like tuberculosis, measles, polio, and SARS were successfully eradicated through public immunisation programmes. As DeStefano et al. (2019) correctly note, "vaccines have been so successful that many people today have never seen or have no direct knowledge of the diseases that vaccines prevented" (p. 726). As such, vaccination is hence considered the most effective medical intervention to reduce death and morbidity caused by infectious diseases (Delany, Rappuoli, & De Gregorio, 2014). Major milestones in the development of vaccinology have seen enhanced immunity against diseases. However, despite of the progress, vaccines are not free from controversies. Vaccines attract public debate and polarization around the medical, ethical, and legal issues related to the vaccine. There are several grounds for these controversies and contests that provide vital breeding grounds for misinformation.

One area of contestation surrounds issues of scientific and epistemic uncertainty. Vaccines are surrounded by a lot of scientific uncertainty on vaccine components, testing, and side effects. Concerns about vaccine safety lead to fear, scepticism, and rejection of vaccines. The public wants to know that the vaccines have been developed in ethical ways; that they pose minimum health risk; and that they achieve what they seek to do. The public needs assurances from scientific communities and more fundamentally that information should come from trusted sources. Trust is the basis upon which an individual submits himself/herself for inoculation. Trust in sources becomes a predicator of what the public exposed to that information believes and translates it into action, where only three options are available: accept, decline, or wait. Previous research shows that trust in scientific sources is an important factor in the public's relationship with science during controversial events (Entradas, 2021). It is natural therefore that the public actively seeks information about the scientific facts of the vaccine before committing oneself. They turn to different sources of information and social networks in search of scientific news and health information. In this broad spectrum of sources, one finds official sources, scientific journals, mainstream media, and an endless list of other sources keen to provide their views on vaccines.

Pro- and anti-vaccine groups converge in these different arenas to promote their views. Scientific sources such as medical doctors and scientists are found across the spectrum. Bioethical issues arouse public debate. Safety and necessity concerns create a perfect storm for misinformation, disinformation, and malinformation. Anti-vaxxers use scientific arguments to challenge the safety of vaccines. As Larsson (2020) notes, most of those who promote anti-vaccination agenda claim vaccines to be more dangerous than the disease. COVID-19 anti-vaxxers use the same arguments from 135 years ago.[12],[13] During the COVID-19 pandemic, anti-vaccination social media accounts were proliferating online, threatening to further escalate vaccine hesitancy related to the COVID-19 vaccine (Hernandez, Hagen, Walker, O'Leary, & Lengacher, 2021). Controversies regarding vaccinations are not new; they accompany virtually every vaccine. Infodemics about the vaccine can mislead the public to believe that a vaccine might be harmful. Much of this belief stems from inaccurate scientific information sourced from the internet sources and social media.

Political Misinformation

Political misinformation relates to government, politicians, and their intentions. This type of misinformation bordered on whether governments could be trusted to deliver safe vaccinations. In most countries, leaders took the vaccines live on television, in a quest to show that the vaccines were indeed safe. Notable leaders like US President Biden took their inoculations live on television. Other leaders openly cast doubts on the vaccinations, and politicized them. The late Tanzanian President Magufuli provoked criticism when he claimed that foreign vaccines were dangerous while urging Tanzanians to embrace natural remedies, including steam inhalation.[14]

Combating the Infodemic

The coronavirus pandemic saw a huge surge in misinformation, disinformation, malinformation, fake news, and conspiracy theories that threatened the effective management of the crisis. These information disorders predate the COVID-19 pandemic. Information disorders have increased tremendously in tandem with the increased uptake of social media and digital communications. Disinformation and misinformation have been noted in politics, business, and various other social issues. Many institutions – governments, NGOs (non-governmental organizations), media organizations, and social media platforms have been working on measures to curb the misinformation discourses.

One way in which countries have responded to information disorders during the pandemic has been through the promulgation of new regulations and laws (including emergency regulations) or through the amendment of existing ones. The COVID-19 infodemic saw several countries, authoritarian and democratic governments alike, adopting new regulatory mechanisms. During an extraordinary crisis like the COVID-19 pandemic, governments are forced to resort to severe and even draconian legal measures in their quest to protect their citizens. Yadav et al. (2021) note that countries have more than 100 laws on the books to combat misinformation, and that since 2019, at least 32 laws have been proposed, amended, or implemented to tackle misinformation. These countries include Zimbabwe, Hungary, Jordan, Algeria, Turkey, India, Pakistan, and Tunisia. These legal measures target different aspects of misinformation. For example, the law in Zimbabwe (2020) seeks to reduce false reporting during national lockdowns:

> For the avoidance of doubt any person who publishes or communicates false news about any public officer, official or enforcement officer involved with enforcing or implementing the national lockdown in his or her capacity as such, or about any private individual that has the effect of prejudicing the State's enforcement of the national lockdown.

However, instead of focusing on general communication of false news, the law seems focused on shielding public officers during the lockdown. The Hungarian Law on Protection against the Coronavirus imposes a five-year prison sentence for anyone publishing false information, while in other countries existing criminal laws were used to detain people who reportedly spread false information on social media. In Turkey, Law No.5651 on Regulating Internet Publications and Combating Crimes Committed by Means of Such Publications[15] requires foreign social network providers, whose services are accessed from Turkey more than one million times a day, to have a local representatives whose mandate was to store the data and to remove or make inaccessible certain content.

Promulgation of laws, regulations and emergency laws, in several countries indirectly curtailed other constitutional rights such as freedom of speech, assembly, and movement. However, not all the regulatory measures were well intentioned to reduce misinformation and disinformation. In authoritarian countries, some of these measures had other motives of punishing general dissent and restricting freedom of expression. Yadav et al. (2021) note how in countries, such as Pakistani, laws have been used to target journalists during the pandemic. In one case, two Pakistani journalists were allegedly tortured by the paramilitary force for their reporting on poor conditions at a coronavirus quarantine centre near the Afghan border.[16] In certain instances, journalists have been accused of spreading false news or causing alarm in their coverage. Cosentino (2021) notes how Egypt experienced a recrudescence of censorship and limitations to freedom of expression during the COVID-19 pandemic. She argues that in the case, "the health crisis had a negative impact for some of the country's most essential economic sectors, such as tourism, but it also presented the government with the opportunity to strengthen its authoritarian grip" (p. 208). While upholding a narrative of combating the infodemic for the sake of effective management of the disease, the Egyptian government cracked down on critical voices and arrested journalists, social media users, and medical personnel on the pretext that they were spreading false information. The dilemma, in this case, is that the medical personnel, who complain in public that the authorities are failing to supply them with adequate Personal Protective Equipment, can be construed as undermining public leadership.

While legal measures to combat information during the pandemic are deemed necessary to counter the negative impact of information disorders on government risk and communication messages, authoritarian governments have seized the opportunity to also clamp down on opposition, critics, and political speeches. Legal provisions alone are not enough to combat the spread of misinformation and disinformation, due to complications in the information ecosystem.

Conclusion

Information disorders have become a major challenge for public health communications. The scourge of the infodemic has been more visible than during any other pandemic before, and much of this can be attributed to the affordances of news information and communication technologies. The spread of various forms of misleading information, promoting unproven treatments, and conspiracy theories has serious ramifications on risk and crisis communication messages. Infodemics and misinformation affect people's understanding of risk, negatively impact on their health behaviours, and increase vaccine hesitancy. Understanding the role of social media and devising effective means to counter misinformation is required for countering infodemics in future crisis.

Notes

1 https://www.ukri.org/our-work/tackling-the-impact-of-covid-19/recovery-and-rebuilding/conspiracy-theories-and-covid-19/ (Accessed 03.11.2021).
2 https://uk.pcmag.com/digital-life/125657/over-50-cell-towers-vandalized-in-uk-due-to-5g-coronavirus-conspiracy-theories (Accessed 06.10.2021).
3 https://www.icirnigeria.org/not-true-bill-gates-did-not-suggest-depopulation-of-africa-as-claimed/ (Accessed 04.11.2021).
4 https://www.bbc.com/news/world-asia-53094603 (Accessed 23.09.21).

5 http://www.xinhuanet.com/english/2020-06/07/c_139120424.htm (Accessed 23.09.21).
6 https://covid-19.chinadaily.com.cn/a/202003/24/WS5e795bb6a3101282172816c2.html (Accessed 23.09.2021).
7 https://h-leads.com/100-fake-covid-19-whatsapp-forwards-that-we-almost-believed/ (Accessed 22.06.2023).
8 https://www.aa.com.tr/en/africa/tanzania-banks-on-herbal-remedy-to-fight-coronavirus/2140066 (Accessed 23.09.21).
9 https://www.aa.com.tr/en/africa/tanzania-embarks-on-steam-therapy-to-fight-coronavirus/2130552 (Accessed 23.09.2021).
10 https://www.nytimes.com/2020/03/30/us/coronavirus-pastor-arrested-tampa-florida.html (Accessed 22.09.21).
11 https://www.newvision.co.ug/new_vision/news/1517283/pastor-yiga-spend-seven-prison (Accessed 22.09.2021).
12 https://theconversation.com/covid-19-anti-vaxxers-use-the-same-arguments-from-135-years-ago-145592 (Accessed 10.11.2021).
13 https://www.texasmonthly.com/news-politics/texas-anti-vaxxers-fear-mandatory-coronavirus-vaccines/ (Accessed 11.11.2021).
14 https://www.aa.com.tr/en/africa/tanzania-banks-on-herbal-remedy-to-fight-coronavirus/2140066 (Accessed 23.09.2021).
15 https://www.loc.gov/item/global-legal-monitor/2020-08-06/turkey-parliament-passes-law-imposing-new-obligations-on-social-media-companies/ (Accessed 28.09.2021).
16 https://www.rferl.org/a/pakistan-journalists-tortured-for-reporting/30687013.html (Accessed 28.09.2021).

References

Allcott, H., & Gentzkow, M. (2017). Social Media and fake news in the 2016 election. *Journal of Economic Perspectives, 31*(2), 211–235. doi:10.1257/jep.31.2.211

Bakir, V., & McStay, A. (2018). Fake News and the economy of emotions. Problems, causes, solutions. *Digital Journalism, 6*(2), 154–175. doi:10.1080/21670811.2017.1345645

Barcelos. (2020). Analysis of fake news disseminated during the COVID-19 pandemic in Brazil. *Pan American Journal of Public Health.* doi:10.26633/RPSP.2021.65

Barkun, M. (2013). *A Culture of Conspiracy: Apocalyptic Visions in Contemporary America.* Berkeley: University of California Press.

Cinelli, M., De Francisci Morales, G., Galeazzi, A., Quattrociocchi, W., & Starnini, M. (2021). The echo chamber effect on social media. *Proceedings of the National Academy of Sciences, 118*(9), e2023301118. doi:10.1073/pnas.2023301118

Cosentino, G. (2021). 'You can't arrest a virus': The freedom of expression crisis within Egypt's response to COVID-19. *Journal of African Media Studies, 13*(2), 207–220. doi:10.1386/jams_00044_1

Delany, I., Rappuoli, R., & De Gregorio, E. (2014). Vaccines for the 21st century. *EMBO Molecular Medicine, 6*(6), 708–720. doi:10.1002/emmm.201403876

DeStefano, F., Bodenstab, H. M., & Offit, P. A. (2019). Principal Controversies in vaccine safety in the United States. *Clinical Infectious Diseases, 69*(4), 726–731. doi:10.1093/cid/ciz135 %J Clinical Infectious Diseases

Dwoskin, E. (2021). On social media, vaccine misinformation mixes with extreme faith. *The Washington Post.* Retrieved from https://www.washingtonpost.com/technology/2021/02/16/covid-vaccine-misinformation-evangelical-mark-beast/

Entradas, M. (2021). In science we trust: The effects of information sources on COVID-19 risk perceptions. *Health Communication, 37*(14). doi:10.1080/10410236.2021.1914915

Goldstein, D. E. (2004). *Once Upon a Virus*. Boulder: University Press of Colorado. doi:10.2307/j.ctt4cgmww

Hao, K. (2020). Nearly half of Twitter accounts pushing to reopen America may be bots. *MIT Technology Review*. Retrieved from https://www.technologyreview.com/2020/05/21/1002105/covid-bot-twitter-accounts-push-to-reopen-america/

Hartman, T. K., Marshall, M., Stocks, T. V. A., McKay, R., Bennett, K., Butter, S., . . . Bentall, R. P. (2021). Different conspiracy theories have different psychological and social determinants: Comparison of three theories about the origins of the COVID-19 virus in a representative sample of the uk population. *Frontiers in Political Science, 3*(44). doi:10.3389/fpos.2021.642510

Hernandez, R. G., Hagen, L., Walker, K., O'Leary, H., & Lengacher, C. (2021). The COVID-19 vaccine social media infodemic: Healthcare providers' missed dose in addressing misinformation and vaccine hesitancy. *Human Vaccines & Immunotherapeutics, 17*(9), 2962–2964. doi:10.1080/21645515.2021.1912551

Humphreys, M. (2002). No safe place: Disease and panic in American history. *American Literary History, 14*(4), 845–857. http://www.jstor.org/stable/3568028

Iannelli, V. (2022). Are there religious exemptions to vaccines? Retrieved from https://www.verywellfamily.com/religious-exemptions-to-vaccines-2633702

Jenkins, J. (2022). Could Novavax win over some religious vaccine skeptics? *The Washington Post*. Retrieved from https://www.washingtonpost.com/religion/2022/02/24/novavax-covid-vaccine-religious/

Kirby, B., Taru, J., & Chimbidzikai, T. (2020). Pentecostals and the spiritual war against coronavirus in Africa. Retrieved from https://theconversation.com/pentecostals-and-the-spiritual-war-against-coronavirus-in-africa-137424

Kligler-Vilenchik, N. (2021). Collective social correction: Addressing misinformation through group practices of information verification on WhatsApp. *Digital Journalism, 10*(2), 300–318. doi:10.1080/21670811.2021.1972020

Kombe, C. (2020). *Herbal Cures for COVID-19 Spreading in Tanzania Despite No Evidence They Work*. Voice of America. https://www.voanews.com/a/covid-19-pandemic_herbal-cures-covid-19-spreading-tanzania-despite-no-evidence-they-work/6189689.html

Lee, D. (2018). How President Trump took 'fake news' into the mainstream. *BBC News*. Retrieved from https://www.bbc.com/news/av/world-us-canada-46175024

Lee, J. D. (2014). *An Epidemic of Rumors: How Stories Shape Our Perception of Disease*. Logan: Utah State University Press.

Leonard, M.-J., & Philippe, F. L. (2021). Conspiracy theories: A public health concern and how to address it. *Frontiers in Psychology, 12*(3007). doi:10.3389/fpsyg.2021.682931

Muhumuza, R. (2020). As Africa's COVID-19 cases rise, faith is put to the test. Retrieved from https://apnews.com/article/virus-outbreak-ap-top-news-religion-international-news-africa-bcc291c6b35e73cc01333d8b5d1af128

Nguyen, C. T. (2020). Echo chamber and epistemic bubbles. *Episteme, 17*(2), 141–161. doi:10.1017/epi.2018.32

Ofcom. (2020). Half of UK adults exposed to false claims about Coronavirus. Retrieved from https://www.ofcom.org.uk/about-ofcom/latest/features-and-news/half-of-uk-adults-exposed-to-false-claims-about-coronavirus

164   *The Infodemic Scourge*

Pelčić, G., Karačić, S., Mikirtichan, G. L., Kubar, O. I., Leavitt, F. J., Cheng-Tek Tai, M., . . . Tomašević, L. (2016). Religious exception for vaccination or religious excuses for avoiding vaccination. *Croatian Medical Journal, 57*(5), 516–521. doi:10.3325/cmj.2016.57.516

Rubin, V. L., Chen, Y., & Conroy, N. K. (2015). Deception detection for news: Three types of fakes. *Proceedings of the Association for Information Science and Technology, 52*(1), 1–4. doi:10.1002/pra2.2015.145052010083

Santos, B. R. G. (2021). Echo chambers, ignorance and domination. *Social Epistemology, 35*(2), 109–119. doi:10.1080/02691728.2020.1839590

Shelton, T. (2020). A post-truth pandemic? *Big Data & Society, 7*(2), 2053951720965612. doi:10.1177/2053951720965612

Swenson, A. (2021). Bill Gates never said '3 billion people need to die'. *Associated Press.* Retrieved from https://apnews.com/article/fact-checking-afs:Content:9917566788

Tandoc, E. C., Lim, Z. W., & Ling, R. (2018). Defining "fake news". *Digital Journalism, 6*(2), 137–153. doi:10.1080/21670811.2017.1360143

Treichler, P. A. (1999). *How to Have Theory in an Epidemic Cultural Chronicles of AIDS.* Durham, NC: Duke University Press.

UNESCO. (2020). *The Place of African Traditional Medicine in Response to COVID-19 and Beyond.* Paris: UNESCO. Retrieved from https://www.unesco.org/en/articles/place-african-traditional-medicine-response-covid-19-and-beyond (Accessed 22.06.2023).

UNICEF. (2021). 5G-The misinformation which is still circulating. Retrieved from https://www.unicef.org/montenegro/en/stories/5g-technology-does-not-cause-or-spread-coronavirus

Voice of America. (2020). Tanzanian president declares 3 Days of national prayer to help defeat Coronavirus. Retrieved from https://www.voanews.com/a/covid-19-pandemic_tanzanian-president-declares-3-days-national-prayer-help-defeat-coronavirus/6187740.html

Wardle, C. (2017). Fake news. It's complicated. Retrieved from https://medium.com/1st-draft/fake-news-its-complicated-d0f773766c79

Wardle, C., & Derakhshan, H. (2017). Information disorder: Toward an interdisciplinary framework for research and policymaking. Retrieved from https://rm.coe.int/information-disorder-report-november-2017/1680764666

Wardle, C., & Derakhshan, H. (2018). Thinking about 'information disorder': Formats of misinformation, disinformation and mal-information. In C. Ireton & J. Posetti (Eds.), *Journalism, Fake News and Disinformation. Handbook for Journalism Education and Training* (pp. 43–54). Paris: UNESCO.

WHO. (2020). *WHO Supports Scientifically-Proven Traditional Medicine.* Retrieved from https://www.afro.who.int/news/who-supports-scientifically-proven-traditional-medicine

Wilson, J. (2020). The rightwing Christian preachers in deep denial over Covid-19's danger. Retrieved from https://www.theguardian.com/us-news/2020/apr/04/america-rightwing-christian-preachers-virus-hoax

Yadav, K., Erdoğdu, U., Siwakoti, S., Shapiro, J. N., & Wanless, A. (2021). Countries have more than 100 laws on the books to combat misinformation: How well do they work? *Bulletin of the Atomic Scientists, 77*(3), 124–128. doi:10.1080/00963402.2021.1912111

Zimbabwe, G. O. (2020). *Public Health (COVID-19 Prevention, Containment and Treatment) (Amendment) Regulations, 2020 (No.1).* (Statutory Instrument 82 of 2020.). Harare: Government of Zimbabwe Retrieved from https://archive.gazettes.africa/archive/zw/2020/zw-government-gazette-dated-2020-03-28-no-27.pdf

11 What We Have Learned from the Pandemic

Introduction

The coronavirus pandemic is a complex mega-crisis that has been systemic, triggering other crises with ramifications across all aspects of society, causing deep economic and social disruptions. Millions of lives were lost due to COVID-19-related illnesses and as a result of pandemic-related consequences. Across multiple indicators, the impact of the pandemic has been widespread. The pandemic has had far-reaching ramifications across the world with a myriad of multidimensional effects. The direct and indirect impacts of the pandemic have been felt across all sectors and spheres of society. In the coronavirus pandemic crisis, no country has been spared, be it developed or underdeveloped, rich or poor, big or small. The pandemic has been more than just a public health crisis. It has been a public information crisis, given the centrality of public communication and information in the pandemic response. The pandemic required sustained risk and crisis communication efforts from public health leaders and political leadership to contain the spread of the virus and to mitigate the impact of the pandemic.

Some public health authorities leveraged their communication successfully, while others failed dismally. The overall communication efforts to mitigate the pandemic have been marked by mixed successes, and muffled and muddled messages that have also contributed to confusion and less-than-optimal compliance with health recommendations. As the world returns to a semblance of normality after the pandemic, numerous questions have been asked about the various aspects of pandemic crisis management. This chapter seeks to answer the big questions from a crisis communication lens. From a communication perspective, what have we learned from the COVID-19 pandemic? What went right or wrong in the pandemic communications? What challenges were experienced during the pandemic and how were these overcome? Is the world better prepared for future pandemics and epidemics? A lot of research was conducted during the pandemic, and many countries around the world have evaluated their responses to the pandemic. Drawing on research findings and evaluations, this chapter provides a synthesis of evidence of lessons learned, focusing on the communication aspects.

DOI: 10.4324/9781003401827-11

Learning from Crises: "A Threat Anywhere Is a Threat Everywhere"

Researchers in crisis communication concur that a crisis is a "tremendous opportunity for learning" (Pauchant & Mitroff, 1992). Crises are seen as windows of opportunity to learn and gain experience. In *Lessons of Disaster*, Birkland (2006) adeptly argues that "even before the wreckage of the disaster is cleared, one question is foremost in the minds of the public. What can be done to prevent this from happening again?" This question lingers in the minds of public health and communication practitioners around the world, who have for two years grappled with the coronavirus pandemic. The possibility of an outbreak of another pandemic or epidemic is present; hence, crises like the coronavirus pandemic leads to efforts to learn, presumably to prevent similar crises from happening or to mitigate them should they occur. Crisis triggers learning and changes through the capitalisation of the knowledge and the experience resulting from these events (Schiffino, Taskin, Donis, & Raone, 2017). As Coombs (2019) aptly puts it, "one way to improve the crisis management process is by learning what the organization did right or wrong during a crisis" (p. 163). Yet, other research shows that post-crisis, learning is a challenge for public organisations, especially agencies which handle health and environmental risks (Schiffino et al., 2017).

As Dennis Carroll, Senior Advisor in Global Health Security at the University Research Co. (URC) pertinently puts it, "The COVID-19 response has shown us that in order to prevent future pandemics, we need to embrace as a core guiding principle the idea that *a threat anywhere is a threat everywhere*" (own emphasis), and further that "only through a coordinated global response will we be able to ensure a newly emerged threat can be stopped before it becomes a pandemic" (quoted in French, 2022). The pandemic has highlighted that an outbreak anywhere in the world poses a risk everywhere in the world. The interconnectedness of the world, through global transport networks, means that infectious diseases can easily spread along the network. Responding timeously to disease outbreaks is a sine qua non for proactive crisis management.

Response to the pandemic by governments has been unparalleled and unlike anything seen before (Fakhruddin, Blanchard, & Ragupathy, 2020). Responding to the pandemic has presented governments around the world with unprecedented challenges, but also opportunities to learn from the crisis. Parallels can be drawn from the previous efforts to contain other natural hazards like SARS, Ebola, and the swine flu pandemic. A unified approach is required to manage public health risks. For public health communications practitioners, it has been amazing how similar mistakes experienced in the past epidemics and pandemics were repeated. An effective response to the pandemic has required leaders to demonstrate effective planning and co-ordination skills as well as the ability to communicate clear consistent messages in an empathetic manner

(McGuire, Cunningham, Reynolds, & Matthews-Smith, 2020). In this context, it has been crucial for public health authorities to evaluate their communication efforts. Evaluations provide critical tools for correction and improvement. They provide organisations with insights into what is working or not working. The COVID-19 pandemic challenged organisations in many ways, and along the way, several surveys have been carried out to evaluate the responses. Evaluations yield insights that should be treated as critical lessons from the pandemic response. The following sections look at some of the lessons learned from the coronavirus pandemic.

Pandemic Preparedness: "Being Prepared Is the Key"

Pandemic preparedness refers to the ability of governments to anticipate a pandemic before it materializes and prepare for a global public health emergency by developing the right knowledge and capacities (OECD, 2015). Preparedness means adequate preparation to manage a global pandemic. Given the global context of the outbreaks and the nature of the viruses, pandemics and epidemics are inevitable. The outbreak of infectious diseases in any country can pose risk to global public health, and hence the need to develop global capacities to prevent, detect, and respond to infectious disease threats. As Youngmee Jee of the Pasteur Institute in South Korea aptly stated; "preventing a pandemic may not be possible, so being prepared is the key" (Maxmen, 2021). Yet, according to the 2019 Global Health Security Index, many countries lacked the capacity to detect emerging epidemics (Index, 2019). This was barely months before the outbreak of the coronavirus pandemic. While governments and global public health institutions like the WHO (World Health Organization) have poured millions into preparedness plans, several COVID-19 response evaluations identify the inadequacies of pandemic preparedness. The Norwegian Coronavirus Commission's report concluded its evaluation on how authorities handled the pandemic:

> The authorities knew that a pandemic was the most likely national crisis and would have the most negative consequences. Nevertheless, they were not prepared when the widespread and severe COVID-19 pandemic arrived.
>
> (NOU, 2021, p. 6)

The report concludes that Norway's public authorities should have been better prepared when the pandemic struck. Similarly, an OECD (Organization for Economic Co-Operation and Development) evaluation report on the responses to coronavirus in the OECD countries notes that pandemic preparedness was generally insufficient:

> The COVID-19 pandemic was not an unexpected 'black swan' event, as most national risk assessment frameworks had anticipated some form of pandemic.

Yet, many OECD countries overlooked lessons that could have been drawn from previous global virus outbreaks, such as SARS or H1N1, and as a result, were not adequately prepared.

(OECD, 2022)

COVID-19 has demonstrated that the world was less prepared than most had imagined (Maxmen, 2021). Evaluations by the Global Health Security Index noted that all countries remain dangerously unprepared to meet future epidemic and pandemic threats (GHS, 2021). It is apparent from the COVID-19 pandemic experiences that the preparedness of public health institutions must be prioritized to effectively manage future public health crises.

Crisis Communication Plans in the Age of AI

Insufficient or lack of preparedness truncated the pandemic risk and crisis communication due to the absence of risk management protocols to guide the pandemic response. There is a need to focus more broadly on crisis communication in pandemic preparedness. Understanding the risks allow authorities to better formulate risk communication messages. Having in place defined procedures and guidelines to follow in the event of a crisis is crucial for orderly risk communication.

Understanding and Leveraging Digital Communication

The coronavirus pandemic has been described as a data-driven pandemic, given the primacy of data in the digital communication spheres. The pandemic accelerated innovative communication solutions, changing the communication landscape rapidly with new digital communication platforms emerging. The new digital platforms are evolving fast, incorporating new functionalities for the production, dissemination, and consumption of information. Communicators need to keep pace with the general developments in communication technologies. There are also huge changes ahead in the digital communication landscape. Autonomous agents, conversational agents, wearable communication technologies, augmented reality, and smart things will undoubtedly affect the future of human communication. As artificial intelligence (AI) gain momentum with new advanced language generation tools such as Open AI's ChatGPT-4, AI-powered search engines such as Bing AI, Copilot, and Google's Bard, new opportunities and challenges for crisis communication emerge. These tools will ostensibly impact on human communications, and hence the need to understand and leverage them effectively.

Understanding the Fundamentals of Social Media

Social media platforms have evolved into potent platforms shaping global communications. Facebook, Twitter, Tiktok, YouTube, WhatsApp, and many others have impacted the ways people communicate about crises and how they seek and share pandemic-related information. In this social media arena, there are little or no filters on the information. Audiences take multiple roles as producers, disseminators, and consumers of information in social media platforms. Technologies, such as the algorithms imbued in the social media platforms, create other dimensions to communication processes in the way they handle data generated in the platforms. Not surprisingly, social media has been a bone of contention for communication practitioners due to its characteristics and the virtual absence of gatekeepers. Problematic information such as misinformation, disinformation, fake news, and conspiracy theories have circulated primarily on social media platforms. Future crises communication plans should incorporate strategies for using and managing social media during major crises like pandemics. There is a need to understand the fundamentals of social media. Key lessons on social media are:

• Have strategies for social media communications
• Train social media managers
• Promote the use of social media in a positive way
• Understand the dangers of social media and how to mitigate them
• Enhance fact-checking mechanism in the social media
• Enact laws and policies that guide social media usage

Revisiting the Role of the Mass Media

The role of the mass media during crises needs to be revisited, given the centrality of the media institutions. These institutions have been central in the communication of risk and crisis communication messages to the audiences. They played an important role in disseminating COVID-19-related information and news, facilitating press conferences, creating awareness among the general public, educating the masses about the virus, promoting behavioural changes (e.g. promoting hygiene), providing a platform for discussions and debates on the pandemic-related issues, and keeping in check the authorities through investigative journalism. Harnessed properly, the mass media is a powerful tool to prevent the spread of disease and mitigate its impact during a pandemic. Key lessons on the mass media include:

• Strengthening the institutional capacities of the mass media
• Training health journalism to enhance good reporting on public health
• Cultivate public trust in the media institutions

Understanding Audiences

Understanding the audience is vital for any effective crisis communication. Another facet of the changing communication landscape is the various forms of audience fragmentation across different media offerings. Audiences are increasingly fragmented within a myriad of seamless digital communication platforms and social media platforms, making targeted communication very difficult. The widespread availability of entertainment and on-demand offerings create unprecedented challenges getting audience attention in crisis communication. Planning for crisis communications using diversified information channels is a requisite for success in future public health crises. Communicators will need to invest in various communication channels to provide information to their audiences. Key lessons on audiences include:

- Audience research is paramount
- Have an audience-centred focus
- Use culture-centred communication approaches
- Clearly define the target audiences
- Tailor messages to the target audiences
- Use trusted messengers

Trust Is the Glue of Pandemic Communication

Trust is an underlying theme in much of the crisis management theory. A significant body of literature in the field underlines trust as one of the critical factors in effective risk and crisis communication. Communication recommendations from the WHO and the Centres for Disease Control and Prevention (CDC), and research emphasize the significance of trust in public health communication.

Trust in Public Authorities

Trust in public authorities has been cited as the most valuable asset in the pandemic communication. The pandemic has highlighted the need for trusted sources of information. In an age where anyone with knowledge can freely disseminate it via the many free channels available, it becomes pertinent for public health authorities to be perceived as trustworthy sources of information. Mistrust in these institutions turns the audiences away to other potential sources of messages. During a pandemic, authorities want the public to change their behaviour based on the advice and rules during the pandemic. The degree of trust the public has in the authorities before the crisis has a bearing on their willingness to change their behaviour during the crisis. Research highlights the importance of trust in people's willingness to comply with governments' recommendations and for the outcome of a pandemic (Prati, Pietrantoni, & Zani, 2011; Reiersen, Roll, Williams, & Carlsson, 2022; Siegrist, Luchsinger, & Bearth, 2021). The opposite is true as a lack of trust between the communicator and the recipient diminishes the chances of message acceptance.

Lessons derived from other public health communication confirm the impact of trust on compliance or non-compliance to public health messages. The report by an independent Coronavirus Commission (NOU, 2021, p. 6), assessing the Norwegian authorities' management of the pandemic, noted that several aspects of the Norwegian society made it possible to confront the COVID-19 pandemic and one of them was the high level of public trust. It concludes that a large majority of the Norwegian population has had trust in the authorities' handling and communication during the pandemic and that "without this trust, the authorities might have found it more difficult to persuade people to follow government recommendations and orders" (NOU, 2021, p. 6). Public adoption of risk mitigation behaviours during a pandemic depends, to a greater extent, on the trustworthiness and credibility of the risk and communication messengers. Evaluations in other countries also highlight the significance of trust. The OECD (2022) report highlights trust as one of the key insights from evaluations of COVID-19 responses. It notes that "more targeted, informed and coherent messaging is needed to foster trust" (OECD, 2022). Trust is not given; it has to be cultivated over a long period before a pandemic strike. Trust is an indicator of the quality of relationships with the stakeholders. Ongoing investment in building trust is essential to ensure that it can be leveraged when required during a crisis. Key lessons on trust in public authorities are:

- Prioritize and manage trust
- Trust can buffer the effects of a public health crisis
- Cultivate trust in public authorities before the crisis

Trusted Spokesperson

Literature on crisis communication highlights the crucial role played by a spokesperson during a crisis response (Coombs, 2019; Liu, Fowler, Roberts, Sayers, & Egnoto, 2017). The CDC's Crisis Emergency and Risk Communication manual highlights the role of the spokesperson. The spokesperson embodies the organisation, personifies the response, and helps establish credibility for an organisation. He/she is the critical human connection to various audiences. Perception of spokespersons' performance and characteristics are crucial during a pandemic, where the audience needs to be convinced to adopt certain behaviours. A spokesperson is the voice of the organisation during the crisis and a credible spokesperson facilitates effective risk and crisis communication messages. However, a poorly trained, unskilled, or untrustworthy spokesperson can exacerbate the crisis. Key lessons include:

- Selecting appropriate spokespersons
- Training spokespersons

Culturally Specific Messages Delivered by Trusted Messengers

The COVID-19 pandemic has demonstrated the significance of trust in messengers in the communication of public health messages. Trust is a relative thing. Messengers trusted by certain sections of the audience might not be trusted by other sections. For example, government spokespersons or high-profile individuals in the political leadership might be trusted by some sections of the audiences, but mistrusted by others. It is therefore crucial to understand the audiences and get messages delivered by those who are most trusted in the communities. This is particularly so with tribal communities, ethnic minorities, and migrant communities who have proven difficult to reach. Local messengers can draw on their local networks and the strength of shared languages to deliver culturally congruent and tailored messages. As Overton et al. (2021) argue, public health communications should be appropriately adapted to individual and community levels in order to gain more traction within targeted audiences.

The coronavirus pandemic unfolded in contexts that are increasingly multicultural and diversified. During a pandemic, individuals need risk information they can understand in order to make informed decisions to protect themselves from harm. While public health authorities seek to reach out to as many people as possible with important risk and crisis communication messages, there are challenges in communicating in heterogeneous environments. Cultural diversity resulting from increased migration, mobility, and digitalisation challenges the traditional crisis strategies and communication formulas such as "one message sent to all via one channel" (Heide & Falkheimer, 2015). Multicultural countries are shaped by many competing histories and cultural values that might even be pitted against each other.

In most communication contexts, there are sections of the population that have proven difficult to reach through conventional communication channels, and hence the need for better cultural competence. Understanding cultural diversity of the audience is crucial for guiding the authorities to devise new strategies and tactics to reach "hard-to-reach" and "hardly reached" segments of the population. Evaluations of risk and crisis communication in Scandinavian countries have shown that sections of the immigrant communities were over-represented in COVID-19 statistics, partly because of the crisis communication failures. A report by the Norwegian Institute of Public Health ponders on the reasons why immigrants and their descendants were heavily over-represented among confirmed cases of infection and hospitalisations during the COVID-19 pandemic. The overall assessment of the possible causes for these discrepancies point to inadequate communication strategies and tactics. Learning points in the report highlight the need to adapt messages to the target group: "An important principle in communication is that it must be targeted and adapted in terms of language, channel selection and content (Indseth, 2021). This implies the need for sometimes extended adaptations to reach different cultural groups. Adaptations can be through finding voices considered trustworthy by the target groups, for example, using religious leaders, community leaders, influencers, and other influential persons. "It is absolutely essential that the sender of the information has credibility with the target group" (Indseth, 2021). For some groups, it is more effective to use oral instead of written communication. Trust-building and dialogue should be the main strategy when dealing with hard-to-reach groups. Recognising the cultural diversity within and between communities is key to targeted messaging.

In a review of the COVID-19 communication in the Australian state of Victoria, the Independent Pandemic Management Advisory Committee (IPMAC, 2022) report also highlighted the impact of culturally specific and in-language messaging to reach diverse and hard-to-reach populations. The message has to be consistent with an individual and communities' cultural values. It noted that "trusted voices such as faith and community leaders, local elders and influencers were as important as medical professionals when sharing information with their communities" (IPMAC, 2022). The use of trusted voices in message delivery gave credibility to the message and was important to counteract misinformation. The report concluded that "future planning of emergency communications and ongoing public health communications should include the ability to support resources, both individuals (including trusted sources) and organizations who have a voice in the community and media, by providing them the messaging and answers they need, in a timely manner, to assist in message amplification" (IPMAC, 2022).

Communications need to consider the social and demographic context of the target audience and groups and adapt the communication strategy accordingly (Lanham, Lubari, Gallegos, & Radcliffe, 2022). The IPMAC recommended the Victorian Government to plan for future pandemic communications informed by the lessons learned during the coronavirus pandemic. It recommended a model that empowers *trusted individuals and organizations* to deliver accurate information (IPMAC, 2022). These are individuals and organisations trusted in their communities. Investing in accurate and accessible demographic information is crucial for future pandemic communication and strategies. Key lessons are:

- The message must be adapted and tailored to make it culturally appropriate and understandable for the target group
- Use culturally specific and in-language messaging to reach diverse and hard-to-reach populations
- Use messengers trusted in hard-to-reach target communities

Messages Must Be Grounded on Reliable Data

Notwithstanding the challenges of obtaining complete, accurate, and timely data during a fast-evolving crisis, messages must be grounded on reliable data. During the pandemic, there were concerns about the accuracy of the data that was used to inform decision-making. Inaccuracies and frequent omissions in data and delays dented the credibility of public health authorities. This was particularly challenging in developing countries that lack requisite structures for data gathering and processing. The use of data to support communication messages should ideally be used in contexts where authorities have the competencies and necessary tools for generating up-to-date data. Key lessons are:

- Use reliable data appropriately
- Simplify presentation formats
- Provide summaries and explanations

Openness and Transparency in Communication

Most literature on crisis communication emphasizes the need for openness and transparency during a public health crisis. Transparency and openness in communication enhance an organization's and leaders' trust and credibility. More importantly, "trust requires transparency, not only through frequent and targeted crisis communication, but more importantly, by engaging stakeholders and the public in risk-related decision-making" (OECD, 2022). Ethical guidance on public health communication emphasizes being fully transparent. "Transparency remains a bedrock value to guide risk communication" (Lowe et al., 2022). Lessons learned are:

- Communicate openly and transparently
- Be available to the media

Timeliness and Consistency of Messages

Research in crisis communication and best practices in the fields of public relations and health communication emphasize the need to be clear, concise, correct, complete, and courteous (Cutlip, Center, & Broom, 1994). Communication should be timely, consistent, and relevant, accessible, sensitive, and inclusive, and targeted and tailored to the audiences. COVID-19 challenged these fundamental principles in many ways. While consistency is considered key to effective crisis communication, lessons from the pandemic show how it was constantly undermined. During the pandemic, there were several experts and opinions on different aspects of the virus and the best approaches to take in controlling and mitigating its effects. Consistency has emerged as one of the biggest concerns of pandemic communications. Inconsistencies in government communications around the world led to confusion, misunderstanding, and despondency. When people meet too many inconsistencies in the messages, they are likely to question the messages, lose confidence in them, and seek other alternative messages. Public health authorities will in the future need strategies to reduce the overabundance of messages and uphold an appropriate degree of consistency in messages. Key lessons are:

- Provide timely messages
- Ensure that messages are accurate
- Maintain consistency in the messages
- Communicate clearly

Two-Way Crisis Communication

Much of the risk and crisis communication during the pandemic has been perceived as being predominantly top-down in nature. Due to social distancing protocols, community engagement has been limited. In their assessment of the challenges, opportunities, and lessons from COVID-19 in the US, Overton et al. (2021) note that engagement with community-based organisations, in shaping the messaging drawing on their unique insights about what their communities needed and wanted to hear and how best to communicate with them, was insufficient. In oral-based communities, community engagement is vital to tailor the messages to the local requirements drawing on unique insight from the communities involved. Properly applied, dialogue-based risk communication can help communities and experts share knowledge and understanding of risks (Ndlela, 2019). Getting people involved in talking about the risks increases their understanding of risks and can help them protect themselves using locally available resources. Public health experts should focus on listening to the concerns of the audiences. Increasing community participation in dialogue-based risk communication enhances the message's efficacy. Key lessons are:

- Enable two-way communication processes
- Listen to the audience
- Show respect
- Connect and engage with the audience

Combating Misinformation and Disinformation

One area of concern during the COVID-19 pandemic has been the proliferation of various forms of misinformation and disinformation in the digital communication spheres. The pandemic has been accompanied by an unprecedented infodemic that undermined public health messages, sowed seeds for confusion, fear, and anxiety, fuelled non-compliance, vaccine hesitancy, and polarisation that sometimes led to risky behaviours. Inadequate public health response provided fertile grounds for misinformation and disinformation. Various forms of misinformation and disinformation impacted negatively citizens' trust in public institutions and compliance with government advice and recommendations. It should be noted that combating misinformation and disinformation is a mammoth task that requires a multi-sectoral approach. Restoring trust in public institutions has been identified as a key conduit for combating the challenge of disinformation in the global pandemic response. In a context where misinformation and disinformation spreads rapidly, trust in public authorities can ameliorate the problem (OECD, 2020). Fighting the infodemic requires that public health authorities maintain transparent communication about the situation. Other interventions in the fight against misinformation and disinformation include intensifying fact-checking services, educating the public and engaging the citizens in a collective response to the infodemic. Public health authorities should build capacities to timely rebut false information. Keys lessons include:

- Build trust in public authorities and the media
- Build robust fact-checking systems
- Enact legal mechanisms and policies to combat misinformation
- Enhance digital literacies

Conclusion

This chapter has explored the key lessons learned during the coronavirus pandemic from a crisis communication lens. The key message is that pandemic preparedness is a prerequisite to effective crisis management responses. Plans provide tools that guide the responses and shape the messages needed in the pandemic management. Understanding the audiences, the communication, and the communication contexts and cultures are crucial for risk and crisis communication. Above everything, trust is the glue that supports the messages during a crisis. Maintaining trust in the communication processes during a pandemic crisis is the fastest way to recovery. Lack of trust undermines messages and only exacerbates the crisis.

References

Birkland, T. A. (2006). *Lessons of Disaster: Policy Change after Catastrophic Events*. Washington, DC: Georgetown University Press.

Coombs, W. T. (2019). *Ongoing Crisis Communication. Planning, Managing, and Responding* (5 ed.). Los Angeles, CA: Sage.

Cutlip, S. M., Center, A. H., & Broom, G. M. (1994). *Effective Public Relations*. Englewood Cliffs, NJ: Prentice-Hall.

Fakhruddin, B., Blanchard, K., & Ragupathy, D. (2020). Are we there yet? The transition from response to recovery for the COVID-19 pandemic. *Progress in Disaster Science, 7*, 100102. doi:10.1016/j.pdisas.2020.100102

French, L. (2022, 31.01.2023). The Price of Pandemics. *World Finance*.

GHS. (2021). Global health security index. Retrieved from https://www.ghsindex.org/wp-content/uploads/2021/12/2021_GHSindexFullReport_Final.pdf

Heide, M., & Falkheimer, J. (2015). Cultural Diversity and Crisis Communication. *Communication Director*.

Index, G. (2019). Global health security index. Retrieved from https://www.ghsindex.org/wp-content/uploads/2020/04/2019-Global-Health-Security-Index.pdf

Indseth, T. (2021). Koronapandemien og innvandrerbefolkningene, vurderinger og erfaringer. Retrieved from Oslo https://www.fhi.no/globalassets/dokumenterfiler/rapporter/2021/koronapandemien-og-innvandrerbefolkningene-vurderinger-og-erfaringer-rapport-2021.pdf

IPMAC. (2022). Review of COVID-19 communications in Victoria. Victorian Government response to the Independent Pandemic Management Advisory Committee (IPMAC) Report. Retrieved from https://www.health.vic.gov.au/research-and-reports/review-of-covid-19-communications-in-victoria

Lanham, A., Lubari, E., Gallegos, D., & Radcliffe, B. (2022). Health promotion in emerging collectivist communities: A study of dietary acculturation in the South Sudanese community in Logan City, Australia. *Health Promotion Journal of Australia, 33*(1), 224–231. doi:10.1002/hpja.491

Liu, B. F., Fowler, B. M., Roberts, H. A., Sayers, E. L. P., & Egnoto, M. J. (2017). The role of communication in healthcare systems and community resilience. *International Journal of Emergency Management, 13*(4), 305–327. doi:10.1504/ijem.2017.087218

Lowe, A. E., Voo, T. C., Lee, L. M., Dineen Gillespie, K. K., Feig, C., Ferdinand, A. O., . . . Wynia, M. K. (2022). Uncertainty, scarcity and transparency: Public health ethics and risk communication in a pandemic. *The Lancet Regional Health - Americas, 16*, 100374. doi:10.1016/j.lana.2022.100374

Maxmen, A. (2021). Has COVID taught us anything about pandemic preparedness? *Nature Briefing*. Retrieved from https://www.nature.com/articles/d41586-021-02217-y

McGuire, D., Cunningham, J. E. A., Reynolds, K., & Matthews-Smith, G. (2020). Beating the virus: an examination of the crisis communication approach taken by New Zealand Prime Minister Jacinda Ardern during the Covid-19 pandemic. *Human Resource Development International, 23*(4), 361–379. doi:10.1080/13678868.2020.1779543

Ndlela, M. (2019). *Crisis Communication. A Stakeholder Perspective*. Cham, Switzerland: Palgrave Macmillan.

NOU. (2021). *Myndighetenes håndtering av koronapandemien*. Oslo: Government of Norway. Retrieved from https://files.nettsteder.regjeringen.no/wpuploads01/blogs.dir/421/files/2021/04/Koronakommisjonens_rapport_NOU.pdf

OECD. (2015). *The Changing Face of Strategic Crisis Management*. Retrieved from Paris https://dx.doi.org/10.1787/9789264249127-en

OECD. (2020). Transparency, communication and trust: The role of public communication in responding to the wave of disinformation about the new coronavirus. Retrieved from https://www.oecd-ilibrary.org/docserver/bef7ad6e-en.pdf?expires=1670859107&id=id&accname=guest&checksum=7BC1F2F4CF74E7C83EF1294F4B26853D

OECD. (2022). First lessons from government evaluations of COVID-19 responses: A synthesis. Retrieved from https://www.oecd.org/coronavirus/policy-responses/first-lessons-from-government-evaluations-of-covid-19-responses-a-synthesis-483507d6/

Overton, D., Ramkeesoon, S. A., Kirkpatrick, K., Byron, A., & Pak, E. S. (2021). *Lessons from the COVID-19 Crisis on Executing Communications and Engagement at the Community Level during a Health Crisis*. Washington, DC: National Academies of Sciences, Engineering, and Medicine, https://doi.org/10.17226/26340

Pauchant, T. C., & Mitroff, I. (1992). *Transforming the Crisis-Prone Organization: Preventing Individual, Organizational, and Environmental Tragedies.* San Francisco, CA: Jossey-Bass.

Prati, G., Pietrantoni, L., & Zani, B. (2011). Compliance with recommendations for pandemic influenza H1N1 2009: The role of trust and personal beliefs. *Health Education Research, 26*(5), 761–769. doi:10.1093/her/cyr035 %J Health Education Research

Reiersen, J., Roll, K., Williams, J. D., & Carlsson, M. (2022). Trust: A double-edged sword in combating the COVID-19 pandemic? *Frontiers in Communication, 7.* doi:10.3389/fcomm.2022.822302

Schiffino, N., Taskin, L., Donis, C., & Raone, J. (2017). Post-crisis learning in public agencies: What do we learn from both actors and institutions? *Policy Studies, 38*(1), 59–75. doi:10.1080/01442872.2016.1188906

Siegrist, M., Luchsinger, L., & Bearth, A. (2021). The Impact of trust and risk perception on the acceptance of measures to reduce COVID-19 cases. *Risk Analysis, 41*(5), 787–800. doi:10.1111/risa.13675

Index

For Product Safety Concerns and Information please contact our EU
representative GPSR@taylorandfrancis.com
Taylor & Francis Verlag GmbH, Kaufingerstraße 24, 80331 München, Germany

www.ingramcontent.com/pod-product-compliance
Lightning Source LLC
Chambersburg PA
CBHW060303220326
41598CB00027B/4216